# Chinese Family Acupoint Massage

Wang Chuangui

FOREIGN LANGUAGES PRESS    BEIJING

First Edition 1992
Second Printing 1994

*English text edited by* Wang Jianguang
*Translated by* Xie Zhufan
*Illustrated by* Li Shiji
*Jacket design by* Tang Yu
*Layout by* Dai Jinghua

ISBN 0-8351-2569-6
ISBN 7-119-01439-0
ⓒ Foreign Languages Press, Beijing, 1992, China
Published by Foreign Languages Press
24 Baiwanzhuang Road, Beijing 100037, China
Printed by Beijing Foreign Languages Printing House
19 Chegongzhuang Xilu, Beijing 100044, China

*Printed in the People's Republic of China*

# Contents

# Chapter One
## Introduction

### I. What is acupoint massage?

Acupoint massage is one of the ancient and unique therapeutic methods of traditional Chinese medicine. It is based upon the traditional theories of *qi*, blood, visceral organs, meridians and collaterals, and is characterized by applying special pressing and rubbing on certain meridians, acupoints, muscles and skin areas with different parts of the palms and fingers and with various degrees of force. It includes pushing and stroking the meridians, digital and palmar pressing on the acupoints, kneading and grasping the muscles, and rubbing the skin, by which the flow of *qi* and blood in the meridians and collaterals will be promoted, the function of visceral organs regulated, and the nourishment of muscles improved. Therefore, it can be used for treating and preventing diseases. It is called "acupoint massage" because the massage is chiefly applied to acupoints and meridians.

### II. Origin and development of acupoint massage

Acupoint massage is an important component of traditional Chinese medicine. It was founded and developed by the Chinese over their many centuries of struggle against disease.

More than two thousand years ago acupoint massage was already being applied in medical practice. As stated in the *Canon of Medicine*, the oldest medical classic extant in China written in the Warring States Period (475-221 B.C.), "Overstrain and fright may cause obstruction of meridians and collaterals manifested by paralysis. The treatment is massage and medicated liquor." It is therefore certain that massage was an art of healing used in combination with medicated liquor and decoctions.

In the Sui and Tang dynasties (A.D. 581-907), along with the development of medical theory and practice, new achievements were obtained in the field of massage therapy. As recorded in the *New History of the Tang Dynasty*, "In the Imperial Bureau of Medicine there is one massage doctor and four massage masters in charge of *Daoyin* therapy (physical and breathing exercise combined with self-massage) and bone-setting." According to the *Six Codes of the Tang Dynasty*, "Massage is used for treating the diseases caused by wind, cold, summer heat, damp, hunger, overeating, overstrain and excessive leisure."

In the Song, Kin and Yuan dynasties (A.D. 908-1368) massage therapy was more widely used. As stated in the *General Collection for Holy Relief*, "Pressing and rubbing may be applied either separately or in combination; all these practices are called massage. Pressing alone without rubbing, rubbing alone without pressing, pressing together with rubbing, pressing and rubbing in combination with herbal medication — each has its own indications."

In the Ming and Qing dynasties (A.D. 1368-1911) there was further development of massage therapy Massage was one of the thirteen specialities into which medicine was divided. Particularly rich experience was gained in the treatment of pediatric diseases, and a unique system of massage for children was formulated. More than twenty monographs on massage were written in this period.

Since the founding of the People's Republic of China in 1949, massage therapy has had rapid progress. Massage departments, massage clinics, massage hospitals, massage schools, massage faculties in colleges of traditional Chinese medicine, as well as massage research institutions have been set up. Various monographs and clinical reports on massage have been published. Nowadays, a number of countries have sent personnel to China to study acupoint massage. This ancient art of healing is becoming one of the necessary methods for preventing and treating diseases for all of mankind.

# III. Theory and action of acupoint massage

Acupoint massage is a kind of external treatment based on the theories of *qi*, blood, visceral organs, meridians and collaterals.

Meridians and collaterals are distributed throughout the body. They connect with the visceral organs (the heart, liver, spleen, lung, kidney, stomach, large intestine, small intestine, urinary bladder, gall bladder, and triple energizer) internally and extend to the body surface skin — muscles, bones, limbs and orifices (eyes, ears, nostrils, mouth, urethra, vagina and anus), making all parts of the human body a coordinated integrity. Nutrient substances such as *qi*, blood and fluid are transported to various parts of the body chiefly through the meridians and collaterals to maintain normal body functioning.

Meridians and collaterals are not only the conduits in which the *qi* and blood flow, they are also important approaches for reflection of pathological changes and transmission of therapeutic effect. By the way of meridians and collaterals, disorders or pathological changes of internal organs may be reflected at the body surface, while diseases of the superficial tissues may influence the visceral organs.

Therefore, disorders of the meridians and collaterals, either due to impact of emotional factors (excessive joy, anger, melancholy, anxiety, sorrow, fear and fright) or due to attack of exogenous pathogenic factors (wind, cold, summer heat, damp, dryness and fire), will lead to impaired flow of *qi* and blood, and hence disease.

Based on the above-mentioned theory, acupoint massage is performed on the principle of integrating mobilization with immobilization, treating the disease in accordance with an overall analysis of the patient's condition and reinforcing what is in deficiency and reducing what is in excess by applying special manipulation and various force directly on the acupoints and meridians. So it has the action of promoting the flow of *qi* and blood in the meridians and collaterals, improving the mobility of joints, invigorating the function of the spleen and stomach, recuperating the kidney-*yang*, causing sedation, smoothing the flow of the liver-*qi*, warming the meridians and collaterals, dispelling wind and cold, removing blood stasis and swelling, softening and resolving hard masses.

# VI. Main divisions of the body surface

If the patients themselves or their family members perform acupoint massage, they should be familiar with the names of the main divisions of the body surface so that they can find out the correct location during manipulation.

The human body can be divided into the following parts: head, neck, trunk and limbs (figs. 1 and 2).

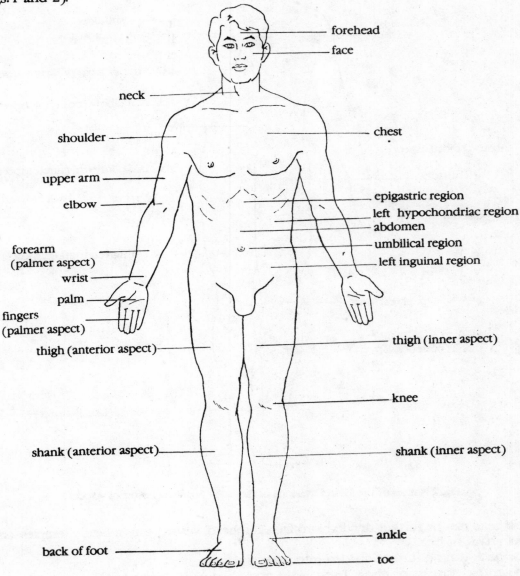

Fig. 1 Names of the Main Divisions of the Body Surface (Anterior Aspect)

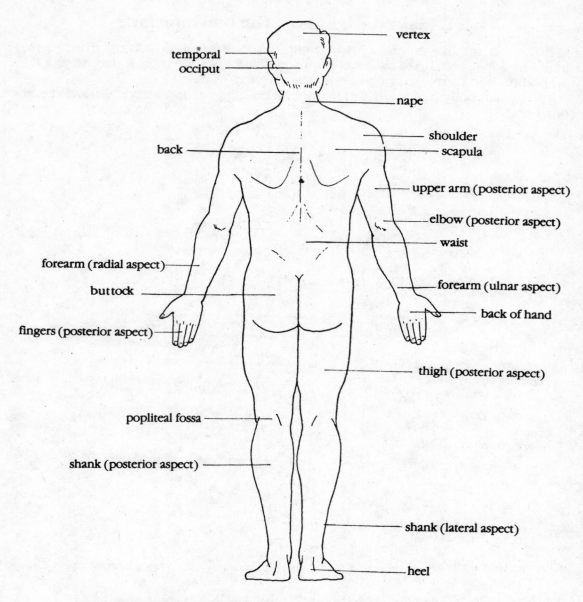

**Fig. 2 Names of the Main Divisions of the Body Surface (Posterior Aspect)**

The head can be further divided into face, forehead, vertex (top of head), temples, and occiput (back of head).

The neck can be further divided into nape and neck.

The trunk consists of chest, back, waist and abdomen. The abdomen can be further divided into the following regions: epigastric, left and right hypochondriac, umbilical, pubic, and left and right inguinal regions.

The limbs can be further divided into shoulder, upper arm, elbow, forearm, wrist, back of hand, palm and fingers; and the buttock, hip, thigh, knee, shank, ankle and foot.

# V. Directions for acupoint massage

Acupoint massage is not only effective for treating various diseases, but also useful for disease prevention, health maintenance and macrobiosis. At the same time, it is safe and simple, causes no inconvenience or pain, and can be applied to either sex at any age. For this reason it is easily acceptable.

## 1. Requirements

Since the acupoint massage can be performed by the patients or their family members, most of whom have little medical knowledge, a definite diagnosis should be made before starting the massage so as not to bungle the chance of receiving other necessary treatment.

When the massage is performed by a family member, that person should take it seriously and do it carefully, focusing his or her attention on the manipulation and constantly observing the patient's response and the change of the local conditions. While pressing an acupoint or performing other manipulations, the force should be mild at first, then increasingly heavy, and finally mild again. However, even "heavy force" should be moderate and no rushed actions should be taken in order to avoid injury to the skin and muscles.

When performing the acupoint massage, both the patient and the family member who manipulates should find the best position. The patient should feel comfortable no matter what position is taken — lying supine, prone or on the side , or sitting upright or leaning forward — and the massaged limb should be relaxed. The manipulator's position should be conducive for exerting force and performing the manipulation.

The duration of acupoint massage depends upon the patient's condition. Generally, each treatment takes 15-30 minutes, once daily or every other day. One course consists of 7-10 times of treatment. One, two, or even more courses may be necessary.

## 2. Medium substances

When performing the manipulation a sheet may be laid on the skin or some medicinal liquid, oil, liquor or powder may be applied locally. All these substances are called massage media. The medium substances commonly used are sheets, talcum powder, liquid paraffin, analgesic liquid, wintergreen oil and Houlou Liquor (liquor which activates collateral flow). The purpose of using massage media is to moisten and protect the skin in order to avoid abrasion.

## 3. Contraindications

Contraindications include malignant tumors, pyemia (pus in the blood), acute infectious diseases, hemorrhagic diseases, open injuries, fractures, scalds, burns, tuberculosis, erysipelas (infection of the skin tissue), myelitis (inflammation of the bone marrow or spinal column), purulent arthritis, severe heart diseases, extreme fatigue or drunkenness. In addition, massage at the acupoints at the abdomen and waist should be avoided during pregnancy or menstruation.

# *Chapter Two*
## Meridians, Collaterals and Acupoints

The theory of meridians and collaterals established two thousand years ago was the summarization of the experience gained by the Chinese people in their struggle against diseases and constitutes one of the important components of the basic theories of traditional Chinese medicine. It has been playing a guiding role in the clinical practice, as Yu Jiayan (A.D. 1585-1664) said: "A doctor always makes mistakes if he has no knowledge of meridians and collaterals."

## I. Meridians and collaterals

The meridians are the main conduits while the collaterals are the branches of the meridians. The meridian system chiefly consists of twelve regular meridians, and Governor and Conception vessels. Thoroughfare, Belt, *Yin*-Heel, *Yang*-Heel, *Yin*-Linking and *Yang*-Linking vessels intersect the twelve regular meridians to enhance their connection and regulate the flow of *qi* and blood. The muscles along the twelve regular meridians in the limbs are affiliated with the meridians, forming a system for accumulation and dissemination of *qi* in the muscles and joints to maintain the normal movements of the human body. The twelve skin areas, including the surface skin and the sub-surface minute collaterals, are closely related to the twelve regular meridians. The skin areas are where the functional activities are reflected and the *qi* is distributed to exert defensive effect.

Therefore, the meridians and collaterals form a crisscross network distributed throughout the body, making the body an organic whole. They are the conduits through which *qi* and blood circulate, various parts of the body (including visceral organs, limbs, bones, sensory organs, body orifices, skin and muscles) are connected and the functional activities are regulated. That is why the theory of meridians and collaterals plays a guiding role in acupoint massage. A good knowledge of the meridians, collaterals and acupoints is necessary for understanding the auto-regulatory function of the human body and for the correct use of acupoint massage.

## II. Acupoints

Acupoints are the sites where the *qi* and blood of the visceral organs and meridians reach the body surface. They are the points of the body surface that reflect the condition of the internal organs, and so the massage should be applied to them. Stimulation of these points by massage can promote and regulate the flow of *qi* and blood in the meridians and collaterals, remove the pathogenic factors and reinforce the body's resistance, reinforce what is deficient and reduce what is in excess, so as to prevent and cure diseases.

The acupoints along the twelve regular meridians and Conception and Governor vessels are called "classical points of the Fourteen Meridians." Each of them has a definite name and location. Those that have not been listed in the system of the fourteen meridians are called "extra points." Each extra point also has a definite name and location. However, there are acupoints with no fixed location or name, which are selected by eliciting tenderness. They are called "Oh yes points."

## III. Paths of the superficial portions of the Fourteen Meridians and the acupoints commonly used

1. Lung Meridian (LU)

The Lung Meridian originates at point Zhongfu (LU 1), runs along the middle of the radial aspect of the arm from the chest to the hand, and terminates at Shaoshang (LU 11). The points commonly used are shown in Fig. 1.

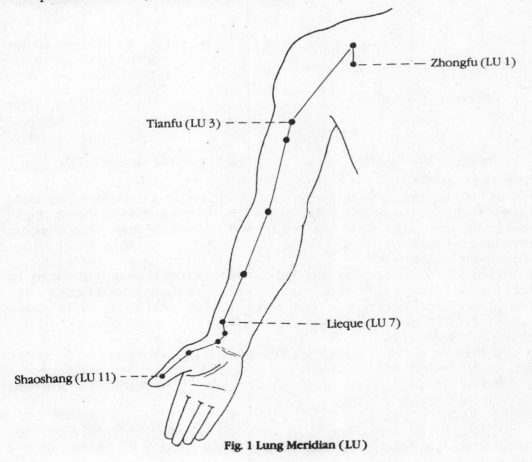

Zhongfu (LU 1)

Tianfu (LU 3)

Lieque (LU 7)

Shaoshang (LU 11)

**Fig. 1 Lung Meridian (LU)**

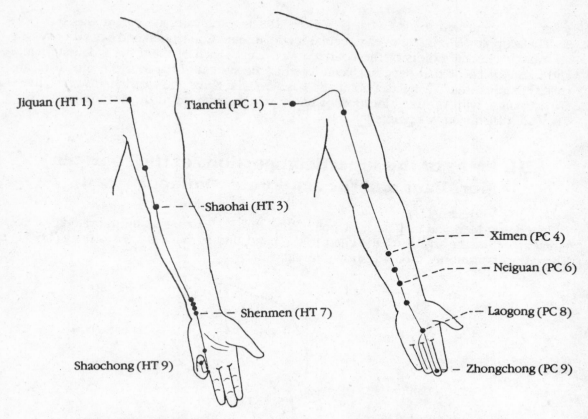

Jiquan (HT 1) – – –

Tianchi (PC 1) – – –

– – – Ximen (PC 4)

– – – Neiguan (PC 6)

-Shaohai (HT 3)

– – Laogong (PC 8)

– – Shenmen (HT 7)

Shaochong (HT 9)

– Zhongchong (PC 9)

**Fig. 2 Heart Meridian (HT)**　　　　**Fig. 3 Pericardium Meridian (PC)**

2. Heart Meridian (HT)

The Heart Meridian originates at Jiquan (HT 1) in the centre of the armpit, runs along the posterior border of the medial aspect of the arm from the chest to the hand, and terminates at Shaochong (HT 9) on the radial aspect of the little finger. The acupoints commonly used are shown in Fig. 2.

3. Pericardium Meridian (PC)

The Pericardium Meridian originates at Tianchi (PC 1) which is situated to the side of the nipple, runs along the middle of the ventral surface of the arm from the chest to the hand, and terminates at Zhongchong (PC 9) at the radial aspect of the tip of the middle finger. The acupoints commonly used are shown in Fig. 3.

4. Large Intestine Meridian (LI)

The Large Intestine Meridian originates at Shangyang (LI 1) at the tip of the forefinger, ascends along the anterior border of the lateral aspect of the arm, travels to the shoulder and neck, and terminates at Yingxiang (LI 20), to the side of the nostrils. The acupoints commonly used are shown in Fig. 4.

5. Small Intestine Meridian (SI)

The Small Intestine Meridian originates at Shaoze (SI 1) at the root of nail of the little finger, ascends from the hand to the head along the ulnar aspect of the lateral surface of

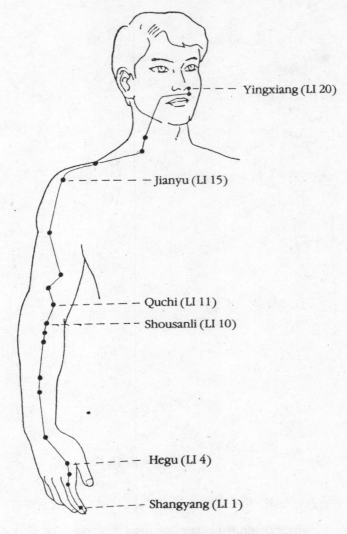

Fig. 4 Large Intestine Meridian (LI)

the arm to the neck, and terminates at Tinggong (SI 19) in front of the ear. The acupoints commonly used are shown in Fig. 5.

6. Triple Energizer Meridian (TE)

The Triple Energizer Meridian originates at Guanchong (TE 1) on the ulnar aspect of the end of the ring finger, ascends from the hand to the head along the medial aspect of the lateral surface of the arm, the lateral aspect of the neck, behind the ear and across the temporal regions, and terminates at Sizhukong (TE 23) at the lateral end of the eyebrow. The acupoints commonly used are shown in Fig. 6.

7. Spleen Meridian (SP)

The Spleen Meridian originates at Yinbai (SP 1) on the inner aspect of the big toe, travels

9

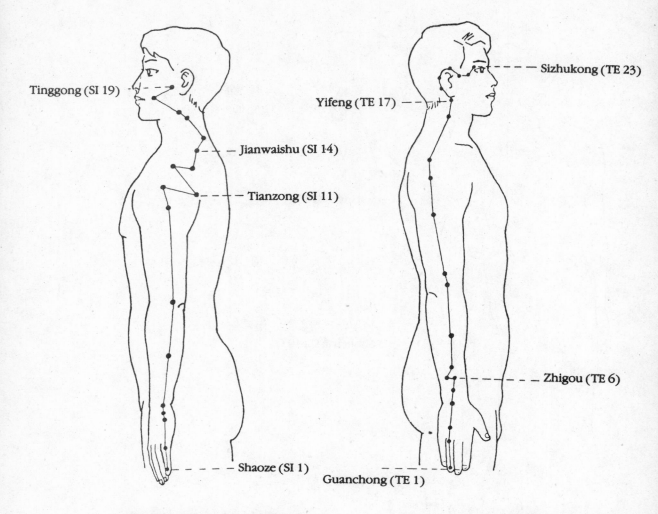

Tinggong (SI 19)

Jianwaishu (SI 14)

Tianzong (SI 11)

Shaoze (SI 1)

Sizhukong (TE 23)

Yifeng (TE 17)

Zhigou (TE 6)

Guanchong (TE 1)

**Fig. 5 Small Intestine Meridian (SI)**          **Fig. 6 Triple Energizer Meridian (TE)**

from the foot along the anterio-medial aspect of the leg, across the abdomen to the chest, and terminates at Dabao (SP 21). The acupoints commonly used are shown in Fig. 7.

8. Kidney Meridian (KI)

The Kidney Meridian originates at Yongquan (KI 1) in the centre of the sole, ascends from the foot to the chest along the medial aspect of the leg and abdomen, and terminates at Shufu (KI 27). The acupoints commonly used are shown in Fig. 8.

9. Liver Meridian (LR)

The Liver Meridian originates at Dadun (LR 1) on the lateral aspect of the tip of the big toe, ascends from the foot to the chest along the medial aspect of the leg and abdomen, and terminates at Qimen (LR 14). The acupoints commonly used are shown in Fig. 9.

10. Stomach Meridian (ST)

The Stomach Meridian originates at Chengqi (ST 1). One of its two branches courses

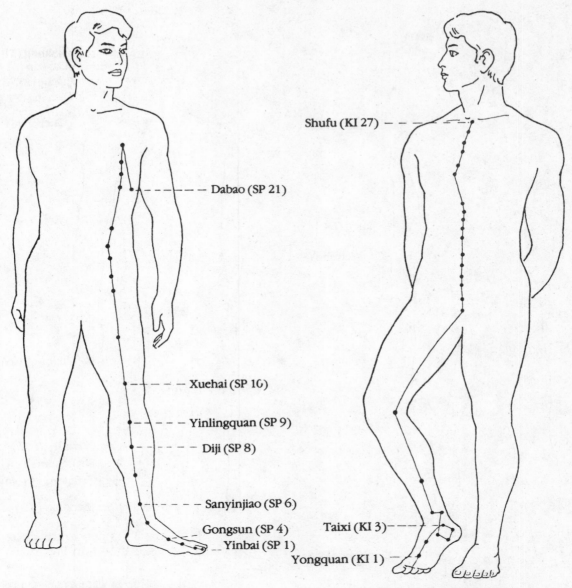

**Fig. 7 Spleen Meridian (SP)**

Dabao (SP 21)

Xuehai (SP 10)

Yinlingquan (SP 9)

Diji (SP 8)

Sanyinjiao (SP 6)

Gongsun (SP 4)

Yinbai (SP 1)

**Fig. 8 Kidney Meridian (KI)**

Shufu (KI 27)

Taixi (KI 3)

Yongquan (KI 1)

around the cheek; the other branch descends from the head to the foot along the anterio-lateral aspect of the neck, chest and abdomen, and the anterior aspect of the leg to the back of foot, and terminates at Lidui (ST 45). The acupoints commonly used are shown in Fig. 10.

11. Bladder Meridian (BL)

The Bladder Meridian originates at Jingming (BL 1) at the inner corner of the eye,

11

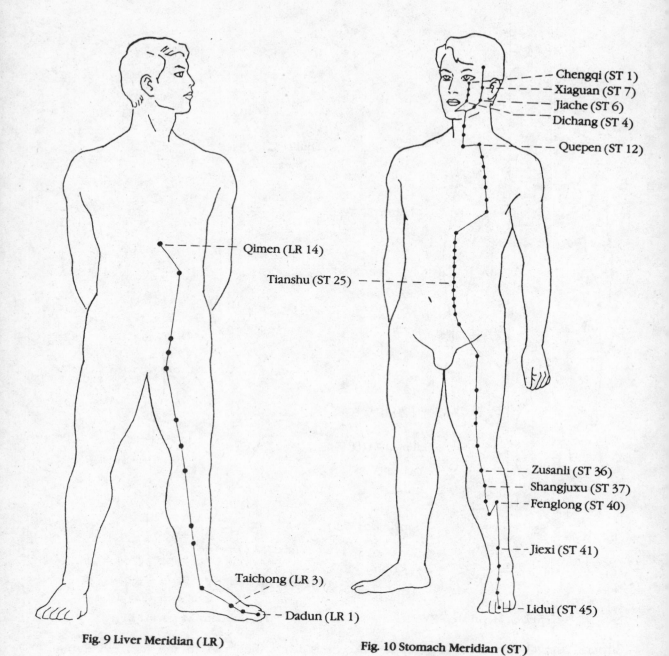

Fig. 9 Liver Meridian (LR)          Fig. 10 Stomach Meridian (ST)

ascends the forehead to the vertex, and then travels downward from the head to the foot along the neck, sides of the spine and posterior aspect of the leg, and terminates at Zhiyin (BL 67) on the outer aspect of the small toe. The acupoints commonly used are shown in Fig. 11.

12

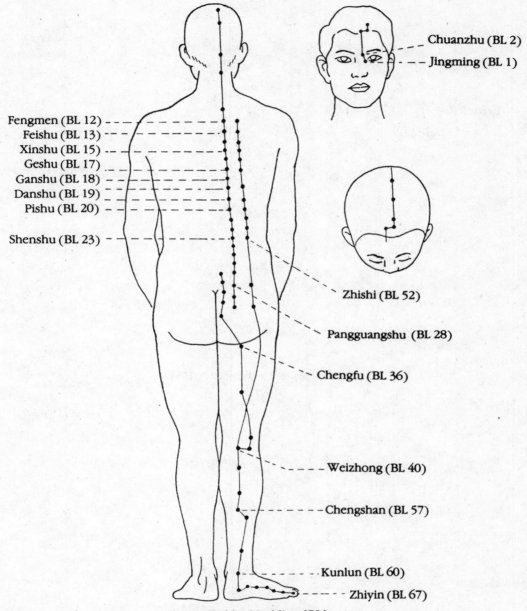

Chuanzhu (BL 2)

Jingming (BL 1)

Fengmen (BL 12)
Feishu (BL 13)
Xinshu (BL 15)
Geshu (BL 17)
Ganshu (BL 18)
Danshu (BL 19)
Pishu (BL 20)

Shenshu (BL 23)

Zhishi (BL 52)

Pangguangshu (BL 28)

Chengfu (BL 36)

Weizhong (BL 40)

Chengshan (BL 57)

Kunlun (BL 60)

Zhiyin (BL 67)

**Fig. 11 Bladder Meridian (BL)**

## 12. Gallbladder Meridian (GB)

The Gallbladder Meridian originates at Tongziliao (GB 1) at the outer canthus, courses behind the ear and along the neck down to the foot along the flank, waist and lateral aspect of the leg, and terminates at Zuqiaoyin (GB 44) on the outer aspect of the fourth toe. The acupoints commonly used are shown in Fig. 12.

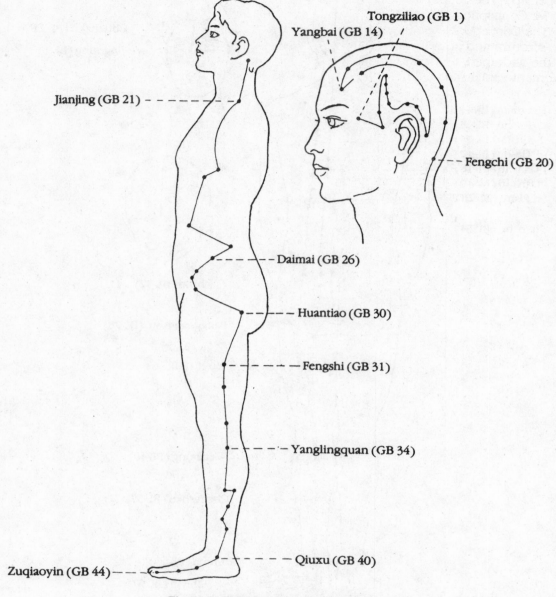

Jianjing (GB 21)

Tongziliao (GB 1)

Yangbai (GB 14)

Fengchi (GB 20)

Daimai (GB 26)

Huantiao (GB 30)

Fengshi (GB 31)

Yanglingquan (GB 34)

Qiuxu (GB 40)

Zuqiaoyin (GB 44)

**Fig. 12 Gallbladder Meridian (GB)**

## 13. Governor Vessel (GV)

The Governor Vessel originates at Changqiang (GV 1) at the lower end of the spine, ascends the back along the midline of the back, to the neck and over the midvertex, and then descends the midline of the forehead, terminating at Yinjiao (GV 28), a point between the upper lip and the upper gum in the labial frenum (the fold of skin that supports the upper lip). The acupoints commonly used are shown in Fig. 13.

14. Conception Vessel (CV)

The Conception Vessel originates at Huiyin (CV 1) in the centre of perineum (between the scrotum and anus in males, and vulva and anus in females), ascends along the midline of the abdomen, chest and neck, and terminates at Chengjiang (CV 24), the midpoint of the mentolabial sulcus. The acupoints commonly used are shown in Fig. 14.

## IV. Location of acupoints

Correct location of acupoints is of importance for obtaining a satisfactory effect from acupoint massage. Therefore, those who perform the acupoint massage should be familiar with the location of the selected acupoints and know how to locate them. The following three ways of location are commonly used.

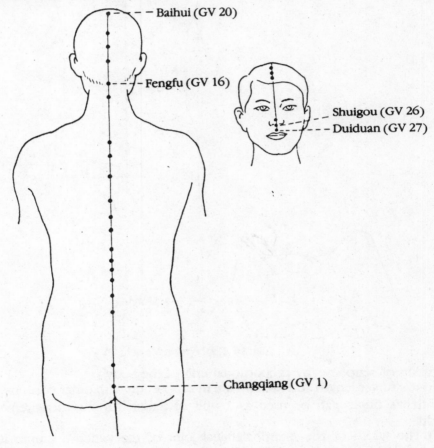

Fig. 13 Governor Vessel (GV)

15

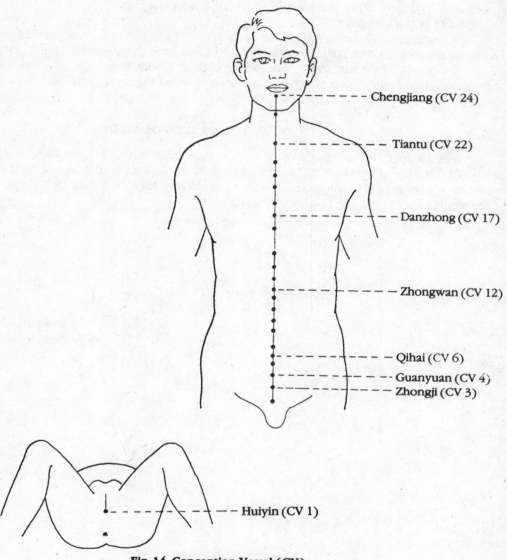

Chengjiang (CV 24)

Tiantu (CV 22)

Danzhong (CV 17)

Zhongwan (CV 12)

Qihai (CV 6)
Guanyuan (CV 4)
Zhongji (CV 3)

Huiyin (CV 1)

**Fig. 14 Conception Vessel (CV)**

1. Location of acupoints by proportional unit of the body

Since one's finger length and breadth are in proportion with other portions of the body, the patient's finger can be used as a unit of length for the measurement of acupoint location.

(1) The width of the interphalangeal joint of the patient's thumb is taken as one corresponding body unit, *cun* (fig. 15).

(2) The breadth of the middle segments of the index and middle fingers together is 1.5 *cun* (fig. 16).

16

(3) The breadth of the middle segments of the index, middle, ring and little fingers together is 3 *cun* (fig. 17).

2. Location of acupoints by bone-length measurement

The location of acupoints is measured by virtue of the length of equally divided portions of a particular part of the patient's body, no matter whether the patient is male or female, old or young, tall or short, obese or lean.

(1) The distance from the centre of the sternum to the centre of the umbilicus is 8 *cun*.

(2) The distance from the centre of the umbilicus to the upper margin of the pubic bone is 5 *cun*.

(3) The distance from the anterior fold of the armpit to the transverse fold of the elbow is 9 *cun*.

(4) The distance from the transverse fold of the elbow to the transverse fold of wrist is 12 *cun*.

(5) The distance from the greater trochanter to the inferior border of the patella (kneecap) is 19 *cun*.

(6) The distance from the inferior border of the kneecap to the tip of lateral malleolus (ankle bone) is 16 *cun*.

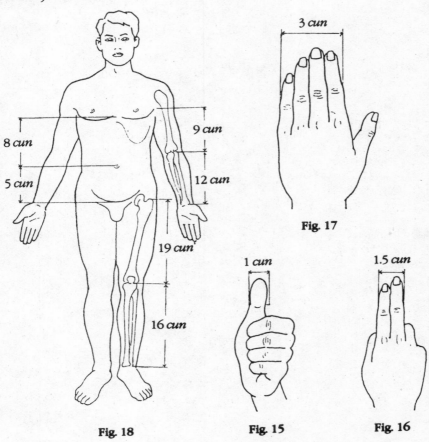

Fig. 18

Fig. 17

Fig. 15

Fig. 16

### 3. Location of acupoints by means of the landmarks of the body surface

Acupoints can be located with the help of the natural landmarks of the body surface, for example, to locate Danzhong (CV 17) at the midpoint between the two nipples; to locate Yintang (EX-HN 3) at the midpoint between the eyebrows; to locate Chuanzhu (BL 2) in the depression at the medial end of the eyebrow; to locate Baihui (GV 20) at the midpoint of the line extending over the vertex joining the tops of the ears; to locate Quchi (LI 11) at the lateral end of the elbow crease; and to locate Fengshi (GB 31) at the point where the tip of the middle finger touches the thigh when in the standing position.

# *Chapter Three*
## Manipulation

Manipulation is of vital importance in acupoint massage. Correct manipulation is always necessary for a successful acupoint massage. Anybody who practises massage must learn with unfailing assiduity and make him or her master of the various manipulations. The manipulation should be lasting, energetic, even and gentle, so that it can be "penetrating." "Lasting" means that the manipulation should be continued for a considerable period of time. "Energetic" means that the manipulation should be done with adequate force which can be varied in accordance with the patient's constitution, the disease condition, the location and requirement of massage. "Even" means that the manipulation should be rhythmic with appropriate speed and force. "Gentle" means that the manipulation should be by no means rough or violent and the change of manipulation should be natural.

The above four points are closely related and supplementary to each other, the overall objective being strength as well as gentleness in manipulation which can be skilfully changed in different conditions for preventive and curative purposes.

## I. Pressing

Method: Press with the palm, finger or elbow at a certain site of the selected meridian or acupoint on the patient's body surface, gradually increase the pressure and retain it.

1. Palmar pressing    Press with the whole palm or the heel of the palm of one hand or two overlapping hands. When pressing the patient's back, gradually move the palm(s) downward or upward repeatedly. When pressing the abdomen, the force should be steady and gentle without any violent action, and the pressure should be synchronized with the patient's respiration, i.e., press the abdomen while the patient exhales and release the pressure while the patient inhales (fig. 1).

2. Digital pressing    Press with the tip of the thumb, index finger or middle finger or with the knuckle. Increase the force to the point that the patient feels distension or tingle (fig. 2).

3. Cubital pressing    Press with the point of a bent elbow (fig. 3).

Site: Palmar pressing can be used for any part of the body; digital pressing is often applied to regular acupoints or yes points; cubital pressing is used for applying massage to the back and buttocks.

Action: To promote blood circulation, relieve pain and remove obstruction from the meridians and collaterals.

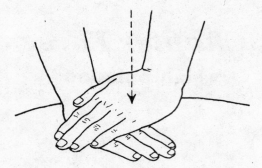

**Fig. 1 Palmar Pressing**

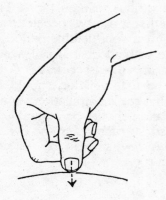

**Fig. 2 Digital Pressing**

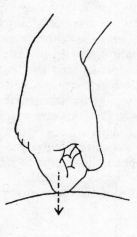

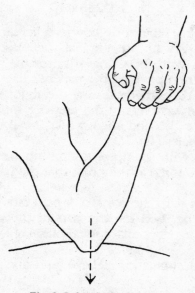

**Fig. 3 Cubital Pressing**

## II. Stroking

Method: Place a palm or finger lightly on the selected site of the patient's body surface. Bend the elbow, relax the wrist and extend the palm and fingers naturally. Press the hand along the surface to and fro in a back-and-forth or circular motion gently and evenly. Light force is applied that can only reach the skin and sub-surface tissue. Stroking is usually used at the beginning and conclusion of the massage as well as during the change of manipulation (fig. 4).

Site: Any part of the body.

Action: To dispel pathogenic wind and cold, regulate the digestive function, induce tranquilization, promote blood circulation and relieve pain.

## III. Kneading

Method: Place the palm, finger or forearm on the meridian, acupoint or diseased area with pressure, and move it around as if making dough.

1. Palmar kneading    Placing the palm or the heel of the palm on the selected site of the patient's body surface, perform the kneading manipulation with the movement of the wrist (fig. 5).

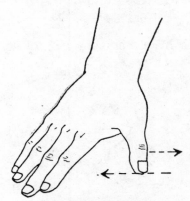

**Fig. 4 Stroking with the Palm**

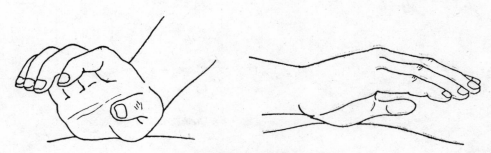

**Fig. 5 Palmar Kneading**

2. Digital kneading    Placing the thumb or four fingers on the selected site with pressure, perform uninterrupted kneading manipulation (fig. 6).

3. Kneading with the forearm    Slightly bending the elbow and placing the forearm on the massage site, make gentle and continuous kneading movements with moderate force by flexing and extending the forearm (fig. 7).

Site: Palmar and digital kneading can be used at any part of the body; kneading with the forearm is used for massaging the back, loins and buttocks of an adult.

Action: To remove obstruction from collaterals, promote blood circulation, resolve blood stasis, reduce inflammation and relieve pain.

## IV. Pushing

Method: Exert pressure against the skin at a certain site or meridian with a finger or palm, and push the finger or palm forward steadily, slowly and evenly with rhythmic movements.

1. Palmar pushing    Push straight forward with the palm or the heel of the palm of one hand or both hands (fig. 8).

2. Digital pushing    Push with one thumb or both thumbs at a certain site or acupoint in a rotary or linear motion with light force and high speed (fig. 9).

Site: Palmar pushing is used for massaging the limbs, back and abdomen; digital pushing for the arms and back for children.

Action: To remove obstruction from meridians and collaterals, promote the flow of *qi* and blood, relieve spasms and arrest pain.

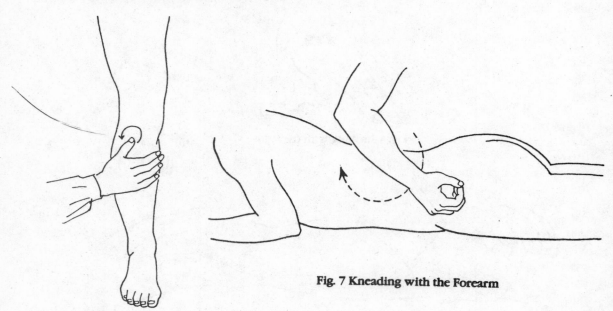

Fig. 7 Kneading with the Forearm

Fig. 6 Digital Kneading

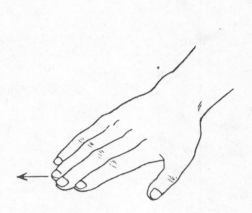

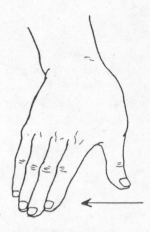

**Fig. 8 Palmar Pushing**                    **Fig. 9 Digital Pushing**

# V. Grasping

Method: Placing the thumb and other three or four fingers on the massage site like a pair of pincers, grip and lift the skin and muscle, and then let it go. The seizing and loosening of the hold should be performed in series and gently with proper force so that there is a sensation of distension and mild pain during the seizing and a feeling of comfort after loosening of the hold (fig. 10).

Site: Grasping manipulation is usually used for applying massage to the neck, shoulder, abdomen, back and limbs.

Action: To remove obstruction from meridians and collaterals, dispel pathogenic wind and cold, promote blood circulation and relieve pain.

# VI. Pinching

Method: Placing the thumb and index finger or the thumb, index finger and middle finger on a certain site or acupoint, grip, lift and twist the skin and muscle with the fingers, and then move the fingers forward successively. Pinching and grasping are similar, but the former is performed with lighter force (fig. 11).

Pinching along the spine    Let the patient lie prone with the back naked and the muscles relaxed. The manipulator clenches his or her fists with the thumbs stretched out and the index and middle fingers propped on the coccygeal region at Changqiang (GV 1). Gently grip the skin between the thumb and index finger, twist and then loosen the hold. Perform the manipulation with the right and left hand alternately. Move the hands forward while doing the pinching manipulation until they reach Dazhui (GV 14). Repeat the manipulation from Changqiang (GV1) to Dazhui (GV 14) three times. Each manipulation consists of four actions: pushing, pinching, twisting and loosening the hold. After three pushes and pinches, lift the skin upward and backward with force to enhance the stimulation on the acupoints related to visceral organs so as to regulate the latter's function. The lifting force varies according to the patient's age and constitution. Use more force for

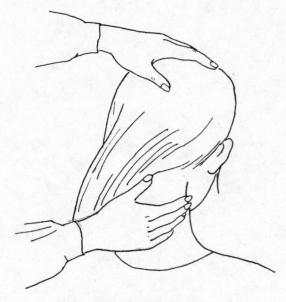

**Fig. 10 Grasping**

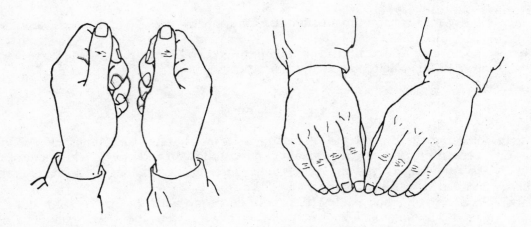

**Fig. 11 Pinching**

older and stronger children and less force for younger and weaker children. There may be an audible "dla" sound during lifting, indicating correct manipulation. Slight redness and occasional burning sensation of the massaged skin are normal reactions (fig. 12).

Site: Back.

Action: To remove obstruction from meridians and collaterals, invigorate the digestive function, promote the flow of *qi*, regulate blood circulation, and relieve spasms and pain.

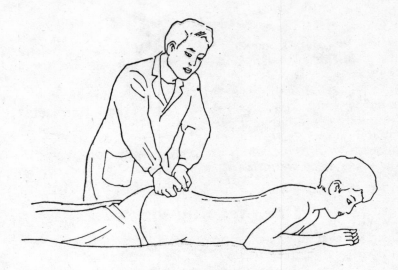

Fig. 12 Pinching along the Spine

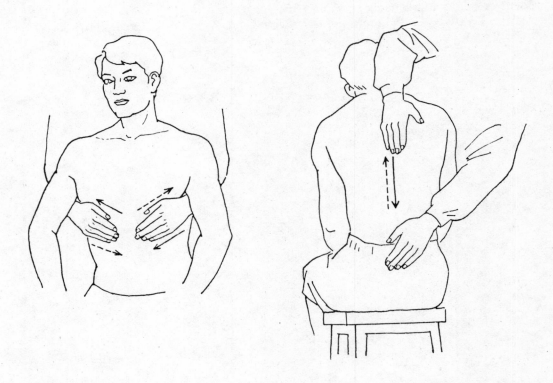

Fig. 13 Palmar Rubbing

# VII. Rubbing

Method: Placing the palm or finger on the skin with pressure, move the palm or finger forward and backward or rightward and leftward swiftly to form a series of to-and-fro movements.

The pressure should be appropriate. Induction of warm sensation in the skin and sub-surface tissues is preferred. Palmar rubbing (fig. 13) and digital rubbing (fig. 14) are used for applying massage to different sites.

Site: Back, abdomen and limbs.

Action: To dispel pathogenic wind and cold, promote the flow of *qi* and blood in meridians and collaterals by warmth, reduce swelling and relieve pain.

# VIII. Kneading-Pinching

Method: Kneading-pinching is a combination of kneading and pinching, moving in a rotary direction with the palm and fingers of one hand or both hands. Placing the palm close to the skin and pressing the skin with the ventral aspect of the finger, knead while pinching at a appropriate speed. If both hands are used, their action should be in alternation and coordination (fig. 15).

Site: Neck, shoulders, back, abdomen and limbs.

Action: To dispel pathogenic wind and cold, promote blood circulation in collaterals and relieve pain.

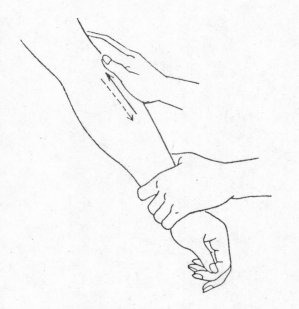

Fig. 14 Digital Rubbing

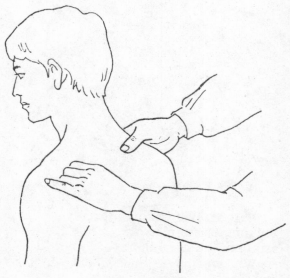

Fig. 15 Kneading-Pinching

# IX. Point-Pressing

Method: Slightly bend the fingers, place the index finger and ring finger on the back of the middle finger, and prop the tip of the thumb against the last segment of the middle finger so that the thumb, index finger and ring finger give pincer-like support to the middle finger for exerting pressure. Quickly touch the skin at the selected acupoint with the tip of the middle finger and press in a fixed direction for a short period of time. Perform the manipulation repeatedly.

The manipulator should lift his or her forearm, slightly bend the elbow so as to keep the operating fingertip perpendicular to the selected acupoint. The force is exerted through the upper arm and forearm to the fingertip. Proceed with point-touching, pressing and releasing rhythmically. Point-pressing is different from simple pressing in the area and in the intensity of stimulation: The former gives stronger stimulation on a smaller area. It should be carried out with caution. The force used in point-pressing may be light, moderate or heavy, according to the patient's age and constitution. Proper point-pressing causes a sensation of tingling, distension or heaviness, usually radiated to the surrounding areas or the limbs (fig. 16).

Site: Any regular acupoint or "yes point."

Action: To promote *qi* and blood circulation in meridians and collaterals, regulate the function of visceral organs, induce sedation and relieve pain.

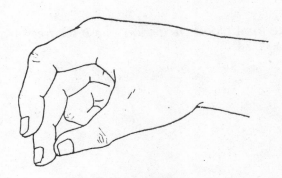

**Fig. 16 Point-Pressing**

# X. Tapping

Method: Half bend and somewhat separate the fingers, support the index finger with the thumb, and relax the wrist. Give quick, light blows on the selected site with the ulnar aspect of the small finger and palm.

While manipulating, exert strength from the wrist. The action should be steady, nimble and flexible. Tap with both hands alternately as if playing a drum. The tapping manipulation is often given as the conclusion of the massage (fig. 17).

Site: Shoulders, back and limbs.

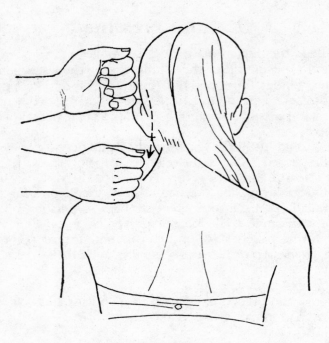

**Fig. 17 Tapping**

Action: To promote local blood circulation, cause recovery from fatigue, and regulate the flow of *qi* and blood.

# Chapter Four
## Treatment of Common Diseases

## I. Internal Diseases

### Common Cold

Cause: The common cold is a viral infection of the upper respiratory tract. It may occur in any of the seasons, but more frequently in winter, especially when the body's resistance is lowered.

Main Symptoms: Itching of the throat, stuffed and running nose, followed by sore throat, hoarseness of the voice, coughing, headache, fever and general aching.

Acupoint Massage: The massage is aimed at dispelling wind, inducing heavy perspiration and relieving the nasal obstruction. It is good for both treating and preventing colds.

[Manipulation]

*1. Massage performed by a family member*

(1) Simultaneous point-pressing of Fengchi (GB 20) and Taiyang (EX-HN 5)

With the patient lying supine, the manipulator, sitting behind, applies point-pressing with both thumbs and middle fingers to Fengchi (GB 20) at the base of the skull in the depression between the heads of the sternocleidomastoid and trapezius muscles and Taiyang (EX-HN 5) in the depression superio-lateral to the outer canthus (corner) of the eye about one minute, and then gently lift up the skin three times (fig. 1).

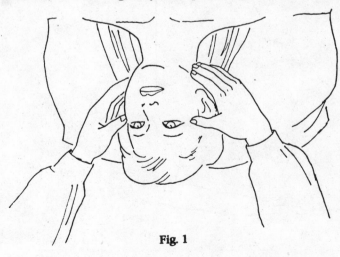

Fig. 1

(2) Tapping on the head

With the patient lying supine, the manipulator sits behind and taps the patient's head with finger tips while the fingers are slightly bent, relaxed and separated naturally (fig. 2).

(3) Pressing and kneading of the back along the Bladder Meridian

With the patient lying supine, the manipulator, standing to the side, presses and kneads the patient's back with one palm or the right and left palm alternately along the Governor Vessel and Bladder Meridian to and fro for three minutes (fig. 3).

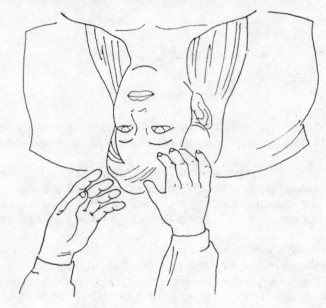

Fig. 2

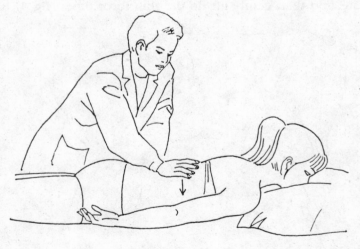

Fig. 3

(4) Pinching and grasping of the shoulder and neck

With the patient sitting, the manipulator applies pinching and grasping to the midpoint between the seventh cervical vertebra and acromion on each side about one minute (fig. 4). It is preferable to induce a feeling of local distension and heaviness.

2. *Self-massage*

(1) Stroking of the face

Taking a sitting position, pass the hands beside the nose, around the eye orbits, along the forehead and near the ears like washing the face. Repeat the stroking for two minutes (fig. 5).

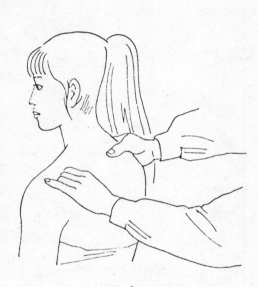

Fig. 4

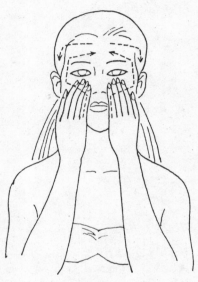

Fig. 5

(2) Squeezing and lifting the nape

Taking a sitting position, hold the nape with both hands, the fingers being crossed. Squeeze and lift up the skin and muscles of the nape with the heels of the palms. Repeat the manipulation for one minute (fig. 6).

(3) Rubbing of the wings of the nose

Taking a sitting or supine position, bend the thumbs slightly and make a fist with the four fingers. Rub the wings of the nose with the dorsal aspect of the thumbs up and down for about two minutes (fig. 7).

(4) Pressing and kneading of Hegu (LI 4)

Hegu is located between the first and second metacarpal bones and on the radial aspect of the second metacarpal. Taking a sitting position, apply pressing and kneading with the right and left thumb alternately to left and right Hegu (LI 4) for one minute (fig. 8).

(5) Pressing and kneading of Neiguan (PC 6)

Neiguan is located on the ventral aspect of the forearm, 2 *cun* directly superior to the midpoint of the wrist crease. Taking a sitting position, apply pressing and kneading with

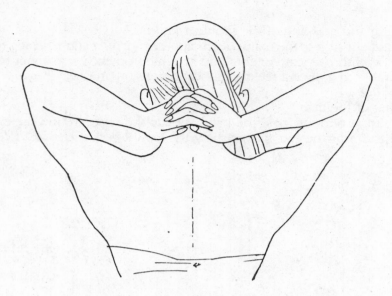

**Fig. 6**

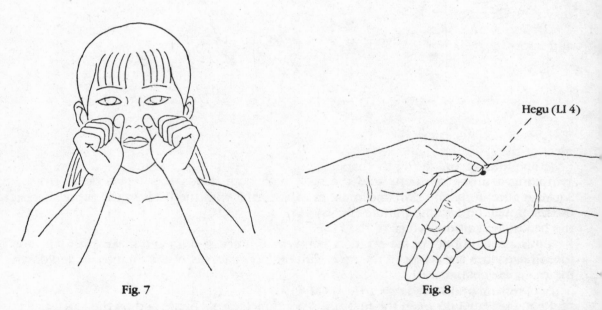

Hegu (LI 4)

**Fig. 7**                                    **Fig. 8**

the right and left thumb alternately to the left and right palm respectively and then to left and right Neiguan (PC 6) (fig. 9).

NB:

(1) It is recommended to do the massage twice a day, once in the morning and again in the evening. Generally, colds will be cured in 3-5 days. On manipulation, moderate force

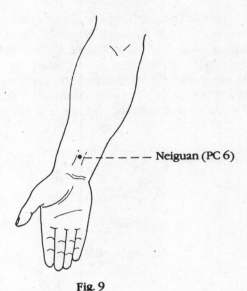

Neiguan (PC 6)

Fig. 9

is preferred; too weak a force cannot give adequate stimulation, while too strong a force may cause abrasion of the skin.

(2) Persevering practice of acupoint massage will reinforce the body's tolerance to cold and improve the constitution, providing prevention against colds.

# Headaches

Cause: Headaches are a common symptom occurring in many acute and chronic diseases of various causes. Traditional Chinese medicine holds that all the *yang* meridians meet at the head and all the vessels connect with the head. Furthermore, the eyes, ears, nose and mouth on the head connect the interior with the exterior. That is why the symptoms of many diseases have reflections in the head.

Main Symptoms: Headaches may be of different character in accordance with different causes. It may be distending in character, localized to a certain part of the head or all over the head. The pain may be dull, stabbing, boring, pulsating or so severe that it is as if the head will crack. It may be transient, persistent or occurring in periodic paroxysms. In most cases, headaches are accompanied by varying degrees of restlessness, lassitude, ringing in the ears, dizziness, nausea and insomnia.

Acupoint Massage: The massage has the effect of dispelling wind, relieving pain and removing obstruction from the meridians and collaterals.

[Manipulation]

*1. Massage performed by a family member*

(1) Pushing of the forehead and temporals

With the patient lying supine, the manipulator, sitting behind, puts the palmar side of the thumbs at the centre of the patient's forehead and pushes toward bilateral temporals at the same time (fig. 1). Repeat the pushing for about two minutes.

(2) Point-pressing of Fengchi (GB 20) and Taiyang (EX-HN 5)

With the patient lying supine, the manipulator, sitting behind, applies point-pressing simultaneously to Fengchi (GB 20, located at the base of the skull, in the depression between the heads of the sternocleidomastoid and trapezius muscles) and Taiyang (EX-HN 5, in the depression superio-lateral to the outer canthus of the eye) with the thumbs and the middle finger tips for about one minute (fig. 2). It is preferable to induce a feeling of

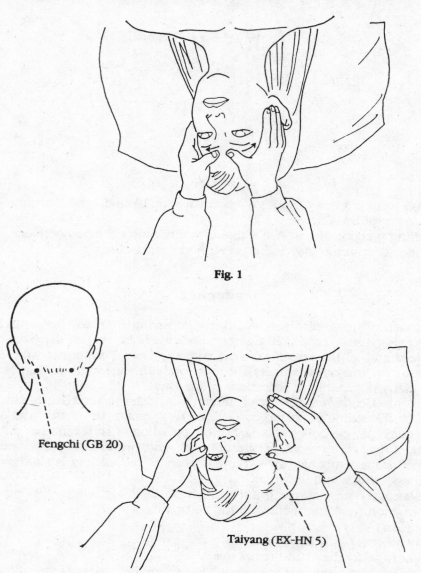

Fig. 1

Fengchi (GB 20)

Taiyang (EX-HN 5)

Fig. 2

distension radiating to the vertex, after which the manipulator lifts up the tissue and pulls it backward three times.

(3) Combing and rubbing of the head

With the patient lying supine, the manipulator, standing behind, rubs the head with the ten fingertips like a comb from the anterior hairline to the temporals, vertex and occipitals together with a vibration action of high frequency (fig. 3). Repeat the manipulation for two minutes.

(4) Point-pressing of Baihui (GV 20)

With the patient lying supine, the manipulator, standing behind, places the right thumb tip at Baihui (GV 20) and the left thumb on the back of the right thumb, exerting perpendicular pressure with the two thumbs at the same time for about one minute (fig. 4). It is preferable to induce a local numbness and distended feeling.

*2. Self-massage*

(1) Squeezing and lifting the nape

Taking a sitting position, hold the nape with both hands, the fingers being crossed. Bending the head backward, squeeze and lift up the skin and muscles of the nape with the heels of the palms (fig. 5). Repeat the manipulation for one minute.

(2) Pressing and kneading of Hegu (LI 4)

Hegu is located between the first and second metacarpal bones and on the radial aspect of the second metacarpal. Taking a sitting position, apply pressing and kneading with the right and left thumb alternately to left and right Hegu (LI 4) respectively for one minute

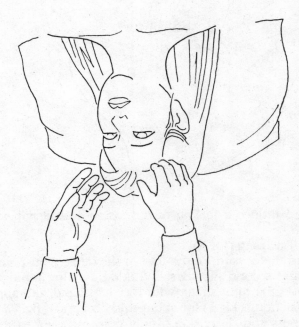

Fig. 3

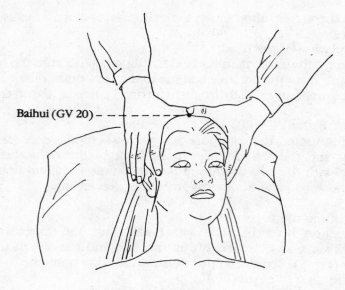

Baihui (GV 20)

Fig. 4

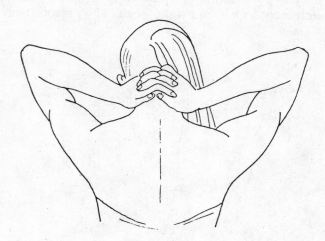

Fig. 5

(fig. 6). It is preferable to induce a feeling of distension and heaviness radiating to the fingers.

(3) Point-pressing of Taichong (LR 3)

Taichong is located on the dorsum of the foot in the depression 2 *cun* proximal to the articulation of the first and second metatarsals. Taking a sitting position, place the right foot on the left thigh. Hold the right shank with the right hand, and apply point-pressing with the left thumb to Taichong (LR 3) for about thirty seconds (fig. 7). It is preferable to induce a feeling of soreness and distension. Apply point-pressing to the left foot in the similar way.

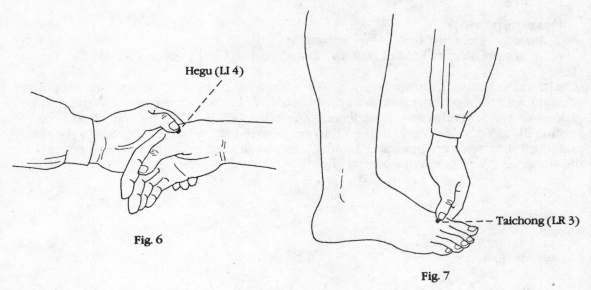

Hegu (LI 4)

Fig. 6

Taichong (LR 3)

Fig. 7

NB:

(1) Headaches may be caused by various factors. It is important to make a definite diagnosis before performing acupoint massage. Acupoint massage is effective for headaches due to colds, overfatigue, neurasthenia, hypertension, menstruation and menopause.

(2) It is recommended to maintain a regular lifestyle and avoid overfatigue.

(3) Appropriate physical exercise and avoidance of mental irritation are also necessary.

## Bronchial Asthma

Cause: Bronchial asthma is an allergic disease occurring in paroxysmal attacks. Its cause is not entirely known. Usually the patient is in a hypersensitive state, and many substances, such as pollen, dust, lacquer, fish, shrimps, bacteria and their metabolic products, may serve as allergens that induce spasms in the bronchial muscles and bronchiostenosis with a group of symptoms.

Main Symptoms: Before the asthmatic attack there are itching in and discharge from the nose, sneezing and general malaise, followed by dyspnea (breathing difficulties), asthma, coughing and expectoration. The asthmatic attack may be transient or persistent. In a severe attack, the patient has severe difficulty breathing, perhaps being able to breathe only in an upright position, and eventually his or her skin or mucous membranes will become discoloured purple. There is indrawing of the soft tissues of the neck, and profuse sweating with cold limbs.

On examination, high-pitched wheezing is audible both during inhalation and exhalation. If the attack is precipitated by a respiratory infection, moist rales are often heard. X-ray examination may show nothing abnormal or signs of emphysema with increased lung markings.

Acupoint Massage: It has the effect of relieving bronchospasms and arresting the asthmatic attack.

**[Manipulation]**

*1. Massage performed by a family member*

(1) Point-pressing of Dazhui (GV 14), Dingchuan (EX-B 1), Feishu (BL 13) and Tianfu (LU 3)

The patient takes a sitting position. The manipulator, standing behind, applies point-pressing with the tip of the thumb to Dazhui (GV 14) in the depression below the spinous process of the seventh cervical vertebra, Dingchuan (EX-B 1), 0.5 *cun* lateral to Dazhui, Feishu (BL 13), 1.5 *cun* lateral to the midpoint between the spinous processes of the third and fourth thoracic vertebrae, and Tianfu (LU 3) on the inside border of the upper arm at the shoulder, 3 *cun* below the armpit (fig. 1).

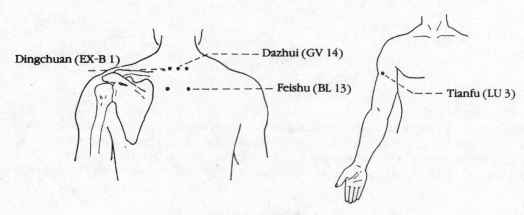

Dingchuan (EX-B 1)

Dazhui (GV 14)

Feishu (BL 13)

Tianfu (LU 3)

**Fig. 1**

(2) Kneading-grasping of the nape and upper back

The patient takes a sitting position. The manipulator, standing behind, kneads and grasps the patient's nape, upper back and forearms with the right and left hand alternately. Repeat the manipulation for five minutes (fig. 2).

(3) Stroking of the abdomen

The patient lies supine with the hips and legs bent. The manipulator, standing to the patient's side, strokes the abdomen around the umbilicus clockwise with the right and left palm alternately for about three minutes (fig. 3).

(4) Pressing-kneading of Zusanli (ST 36) and Fenglong (ST 40)

With the patient lying supine, the manipulator, standing to the side, applies pressing-kneading with the tip of the thumb to Zusanli (ST 36), 3 *cun* inferior to the lateral aspect of the knee and one finger's breadth lateral to the tibial crest, and Fenglong (ST 40) at the midpoint between the lateral aspect of the knee and the lateral malleolus (ankle bone), each for thirty seconds (fig. 4).

(5) Pinching along the spine

With the patient lying prone, the manipulator props the index and middle fingers of both hands on the patient's coccygeal region and pushes forward the fingers of the right and left hand alternately along the Governor Vessel up to the seventh cervical vertebra

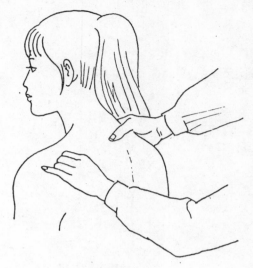

Fig. 2

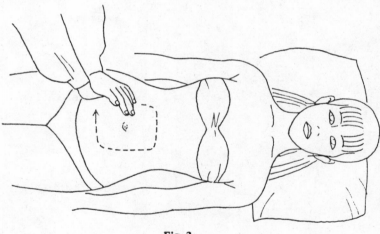

Fig. 3

while pinching. After three pushes and pinches, lift up the skin once (fig. 5). Repeat the manipulation 3-4 times.

2. *Self-massage*

(1) Pressing-kneading of Danzhong (CV 17) and Tiantu (CV 22)

Taking a sitting position, point-press Danzhong (CV 17) on the anterior midline, at the level of the fourth intercostal space and at the midpoint between the two nipples, and Tiantu (CV 22) in the centre of the depression above the upper border of the sternum, each for one minute (fig. 6).

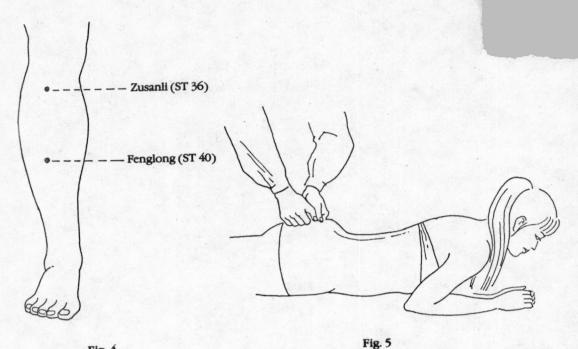

Zusanli (ST 36)

Fenglong (ST 40)

Fig. 4

Fig. 5

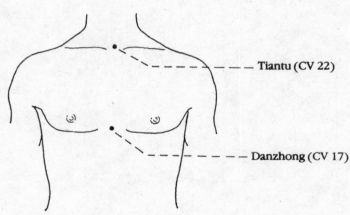

Tiantu (CV 22)

Danzhong (CV 17)

Fig. 6

(2) Pushing of the nape

Taking a sitting position, push a palm with the fingers close together along the clavicle (collar bone), behind the ear lobe and up to the side of the cervical vertebrae, repeating it for one minute. Then push the other palm in the same way (fig. 7).

(3) Tapping on the chest and costal regions

Lying supine, bend the fingers of one hand and close them together with the fingertips placed on one level; tap the chest with the fingertips along the sides of the sternum and intercostal spaces to the subaxillary region (below the armpit) like a bird pecking, repeating this for one minute. Then tap the other side of the chest with the other hand in the same way (fig. 8).

NB:

(1) Prevention of colds and appropriate physical exercise should be recommended.

(2) Food that may cause allergy, such as fish and shrimps as well as stimulating gases or dust, should be avoided.

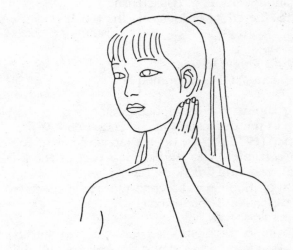

Fig. 7

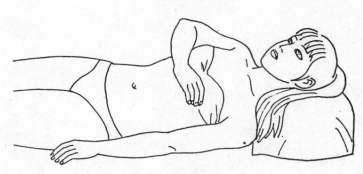

Fig. 8

# Hypertension

Cause: Hypertension, increased arterial blood pressure, is a common disease occurring in those past the middle age. Generally speaking, hypertension can be defined as persistent elevation of the blood pressure over 140/90 mmHg at rest. In most cases, it is related with long-term mental tension or repeated fits of the sulks that cause functional disturbances of the cerebral cortex, especially its regulation of the vaso-motor centre, resulting in

41

constriction of the blood vessels, spasms of arterioles and disorders of microcirculation. As a result, the circulatory resistance is increased and the blood pressure elevated.

Main Symptoms: Persistent elevation of blood pressure over 140/90 mmHg, accompanied by dizziness, headaches, feeling of distension in the head, tinnitus (ringing in the ears), blurred vision, insomnia, palpitation, numbness of the fingers, a sensation of stuffiness in the chest, irritability and lassitude. In a severe case, there may be a sudden aggravation with rapid rise of blood pressure, severe headache, angina pectoris, dyspnea (difficulty breathing), nausea, vomiting, and even loss of consciousness.

Acupoint Massage: It has the effect of lowering the blood pressure and alleviating the subjective symptoms.

[Manipulation]

*1. Massage performed by a family member*

(1) Point-pressing of Quchi (LI 11), Shenmen (HT 7), Zusanli (ST 36) and Taichong (LR 3)

With the patient lying supine, the manipulator, standing to the side, applies point-pressing to Quchi (LI 11), in the depression at the lateral end of the elbow crease when the elbow is flexed, Shenmen (HT 7), in the depression at the ulnar end of the ventral wrist crease, Zusanli (ST 36), 3 *cun* inferior to the lateral aspect of the knee and one finger's breadth lateral to the tibial crest, and Taichong (LR 3), on the dorsum of the foot 1.5 *cun* proximal to the articulation of the first and second metatarsals, each for about one minute (fig. 1). A local feeling of distension is preferred.

(2) Stroking of the upper abdomen

With the patient lying supine, the manipulator, standing to the side, strokes the upper abdomen and hypochondriac region upward and downward with the right and left palm and fingers alternately for two minutes (fig. 2).

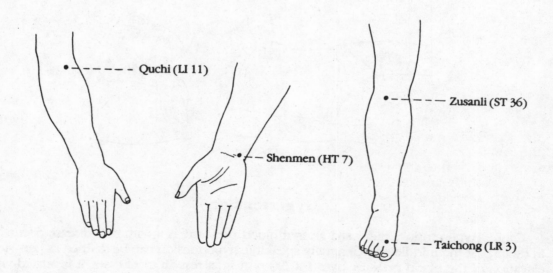

Quchi (LI 11)

Zusanli (ST 36)

Shenmen (HT 7)

Taichong (LR 3)

**Fig. 1**

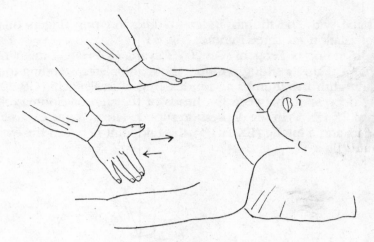

**Fig. 2**

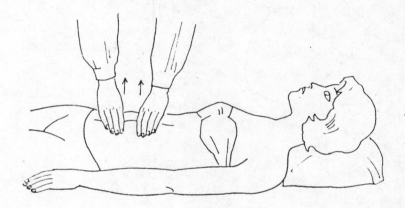

**Fig. 3**

(3) Grasping of the abdominal muscles

With the patient lying supine, the manipulator, standing to the side, squeezes and grasps the abdominal muscles with the right and left hand alternately, starting the grasping from the lateral aspect of the abdomen and working gradually to the medial, and also from the lower abdomen to the upper. Repeat the manipulation for two minutes (fig. 3).

(4) Pushing-kneading of the Bladder Meridian on the back

With the patient lying prone, the manipulator, standing to the side, pushes and kneads the back along the Bladder Meridian between the first thoracic vertebra and the lumbo-sacral region downward and upward with the right and left hand alternately. Repeat the manipulation for about seven minutes (fig. 4).

(5) Pinching-grasping of the upper back

With the patient sitting upright, the manipulator, standing to the side, holds the shoulder with one hand, and applies pinching and grasping symmetrically to the upper back and the nape with the thumb, index, middle and ring fingers of the other hand. Repeat the manipulation for three minutes (fig. 5).

(6) Pressing-kneading of Fengchi (GB 20), Taiyang (EX-HN 5) and Yintang (EX-HN 3)

With the patient taking a sitting position, the manipulator, standing to the side, applies pressing-kneading with the thumbs and index fingers to Fengchi (GB 20) at the base of the skull, in the depression between the heads of the sternocleidomastoid and trapezius muscles, Taiyang (EX-HN 5) in the depression superio-lateral to the external canthus (outer corner) of the eye, and Yintang (EX-HN 3), the midpoint between the eyebrows, each for about one minute (fig. 6).

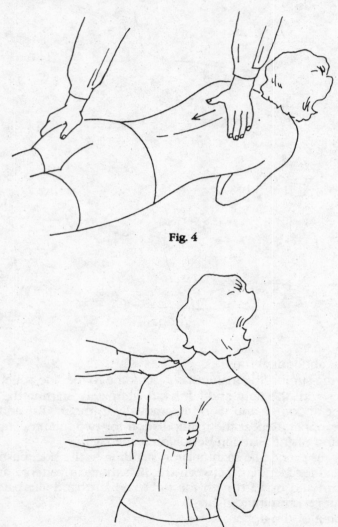

Fig. 4

Fig. 5

44

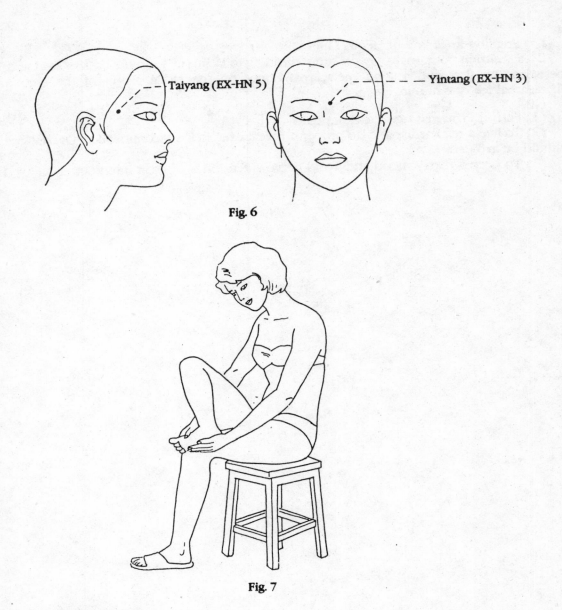

Taiyang (EX-HN 5)　　　　　　Yintang (EX-HN 3)

Fig. 6

Fig. 7

2. Self-massage

(1) Rubbing of Yongquan (KI 1)

Take a sitting position. Place the right foot on the left knee, hold the back of the right foot with the right hand and rub Yongquan (KI 1) in the centre of the sole with the hypothenar eminence of the left hand for about three minutes (fig. 7). Then rub Yongquan of the left foot in the similar way.

(2) Pinching-grasping of the nape

Take a sitting position. Pinch and grasp the nape with one hand, and repeat it for two minutes (fig. 8).

(3) Pressing-kneading of Hegu (LI 4)

Take a sitting position. Apply pressing-kneading to Hegu (LI 4) on the back of the hand, between the first and second metacarpal bones on the radial aspect of the second metacarpal for one minute (fig. 9).

NB:

(1) Perform the massage 1-2 times daily.

(2) To live a regular life and do proper physical exercises is recommended. Overfatigue should be avoided.

(3) To keep a merry mood and avoid nervous tension is of great importance.

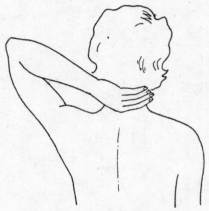

Fig. 8

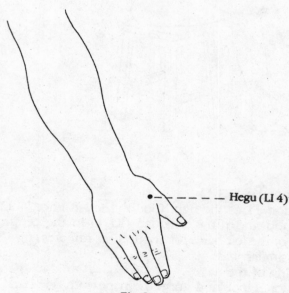

Hegu (LI 4)

Fig. 9

## Angina Pectoris

Cause: Angina pectoris (severe chest pain) is a symptom of coronary insufficiency which leads to transient local blockage of the blood vessels and deficiency in the oxygen reaching the heart, usually seen in coronary arteriosclerosis. The coronary arteries are the main vessels that supply blood to the heart. If the deposits of lipids and cholesterol on their walls cause narrowing or clotting, the blood flow to the heart is impeded and angina pectoris ensues.

Traditional Chinese medicine holds that angina pectoris is chiefly due to stagnation of the flow of *qi* and blood in the heart, pertaining to the category of *xiongbi* (chest pain due to circulatory obstruction).

Main Symptoms: Paroxysmal and transient pain below the sternum and before the heart accompanied by a feeling of compression, suffocation or distension in the chest, frequently radiating to the inner aspect of the left upper arm or the left aspect of the neck and shoulder. It is often precipitated by fatigue, emotional upset, heavy meals or exposure to cold.

Acupoint Massage: It has the effect of regulating the flow of *qi*, promoting the blood circulation and removing blood stagnation.

**[Manipulation]**

*1. Massage performed by a family member*

(1) Pressing-kneading of Neiguan (PC 6)

With the patient lying supine, the manipulator, standing to the side, applies pressing-kneading with the tip of the thumbs to Neiguan (PC 6) on the anterior aspect of the forearm, 2 *cun* directly superior to the midpoint of the wrist crest between the two tendons, for about two minutes (fig. 1). It is preferable to have a feeling of soreness and numbness somewhat radiating to the elbow or the upper arm.

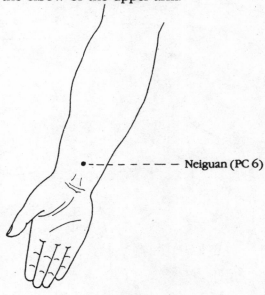

Neiguan (PC 6)

**Fig. 1**

(2) Pushing of the chest and arm

With the patient lying supine, the manipulator, standing behind, applies pushing with the right and left palms and fingers at the same time from the medial part of the chest to the lateral in separate directions. Repeat this for two minutes. Then apply pushing and rubbing from the anterior aspect of the shoulder to the inner aspect of the arm, repeating this for one minute on each side (fig. 2).

(3) Point-pressing of Danzhong (CV 17)

With the patient lying supine, the manipulator, standing behind, applies point-pressing with the tip of the middle finger to Danzhong (CV 17) on the midsternal line at the level of the fourth intercostal space and at the midpoint between the two nipples for one minute (fig. 3).

(4) Point-pressing of Xinshu (BL 15) and Feishu (BL 13)

With the patient lying prone, the manipulator, standing to the side, applies point-pressing with the tip of thumbs to Xinshu (BL 15), 1.5 *cun* lateral to the midpoint between

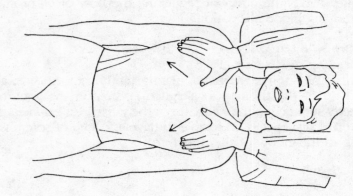

Fig. 2

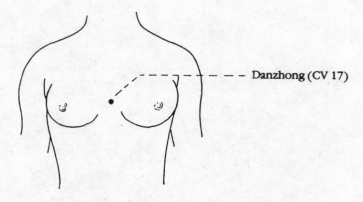

Fig. 3

48

the spinous processes of the fifth and sixth thoracic vertebrae, and Feishu (BL 13), 1.5 *cun* lateral to the midpoint between the spinous processes of the third and fourth thoracic vertebrae, each for about one minute (fig. 4). It is preferable to cause a feeling of soreness and distension.

(5) Pressing-kneading of the back

With the patient lying prone, the manipulator, standing to the side, presses and kneads the back from the upper portion to the lumbar region along the Bladder Meridian with the right and left hand alternately (fig. 5). Repeat the manipulation for five minutes.

*2. Self-massage*

(1) Rubbing of the chest

Lie supine. Alternately place the right and left palm and fingers on the skin with

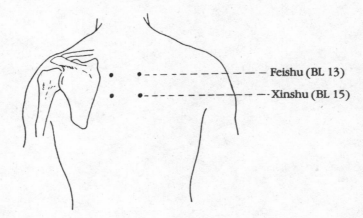

Feishu (BL 13)

Xinshu (BL 15)

Fig. 4

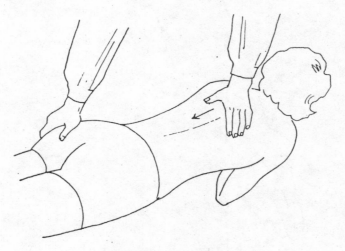

Fig. 5

pressure and rub the opposite side of the chest from the medial to the lateral along the intercostal spaces (fig. 6). Repeat rubbing of each side for two minutes.

(2) Point-pressing of Ximen (PC 4)

Lie supine. Apply point-pressing with the right and left thumb tip alternately to left and right Ximen (PC 4) on the anterior aspect of the forearm, 5 *cun* superior to the wrist crease and between the two tendons, each for one minute (fig. 7). It is preferable to induce a feeling of distension, somewhat radiating to the hand.

(3) Stroking of the upper abdomen

Lie supine with the legs bent. Place the right palm on the upper abdomen and the left palm on the back of the right hand. Stroke the upper abdomen with both hands at the

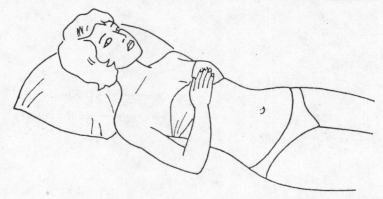

Fig. 6

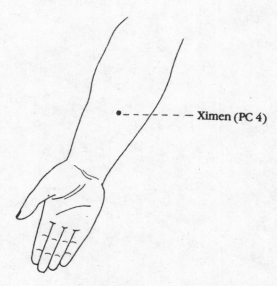

Fig. 7

same time, upward on the right aspect and downward on the left aspect, forming circular movements. Continue this for about five minutes (fig. 8).

NB:

(1) Acupoint massage twice a day in the morning and evening can prevent the development of angina pectoris.

(2) During an attack of angina pectoris, the patient should be kept in bed and closely observed. Sometimes, hospitalization may be necessary.

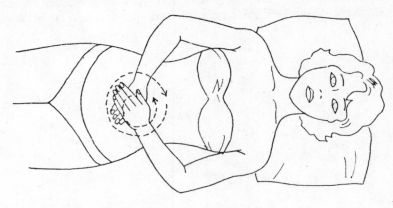

Fig. 8

## Gastroptosis

Cause: Gastroptosis is often due to long-standing digestive hypofunction which leads to malnutrition and emaciation with resultant slender figure, fat deficit and muscular relaxation of the abdominal wall, and diminished abdominal pressure; it also occurs in those with weak and lean constitution and in women who have borne more than one child.

Traditional Chinese medicine holds that gastroptosis is caused by hypofunction of the spleen with sinking of the *qi*.

Main Symptoms: Emaciation, lack of strength, impaired appetite, distension, pain or feeling of weighing in the upper abdomen after eating, which is alleviated while lying and aggravated while standing, accompanied by belching, acid regurgiation or vomiting, and sometimes cardiac palpitation, dizziness and insomnia.

On x-ray barium meal examination, the lower end of the stomach is below the normal with diminished gastric tonus.

Acupoint Massage: It has the effect of improving the gastric tonus and general constitution.

[**Manipulation**]

*1. Massage performed by a family member*

(1) Point-pressing of Zhongwan (CV 12), Qihai (CV 6) and Guanyuan (CV 4)

Wth the patient lying supine, the manipulator, standing to the side, applies point-pressing to Zhongwan (CV 12), 4 *cun* superior to the umbilicus, Qihai (CV 6), 1.5 *cun* inferior to the umbilicus, and Guanyuan (CV 4), 3 *cun* inferior to the umbilicus, each for one minute (fig. 1).

(2) Pushing of the fundus (bottom) of the stomach

With the patient lying supine with the hips and legs bent, the manipulator, standing by the patient's right side, places the ulnar aspect of the right palm on the left aspect of the lower abbomen where the lower end of the stomach is situated, gradually pushes the gastric fundus (bottom of the stomach) from the lateral to the medial and upward to the umbilicus while the patient exhales, and relaxing the pushing while the patient inhales (fig. 2). Repeat this for five minutes. The manipulation should be gradually increased in depth with heavy but slow movements; rapid and violent actions should be avoided.

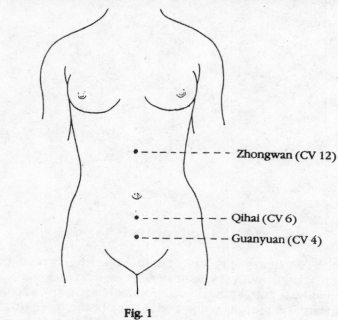

— — — — — — — Zhongwan (CV 12)

— — — — — — Qihai (CV 6)

— — — — — — Guanyuan (CV 4)

**Fig. 1**

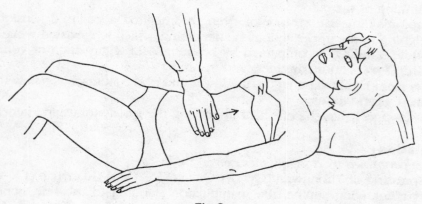

**Fig. 2**

(3) Stroking of the abdomen

With the patient lying supine, the manipulator, standing to the side, strokes the abdomen with the right and left palm alternately from the upper abdomen to the umbilicus and then to the lower abdomen, forming clockwise and counterclockwise circular movements and extending to the whole abdomen (fig. 3). Repeat the manipulation for three minutes.

(4) Pressing-kneading of Zusanli (ST 36)

With the patient lying supine, the manipulator applies pressing-kneading to Zusanli (ST

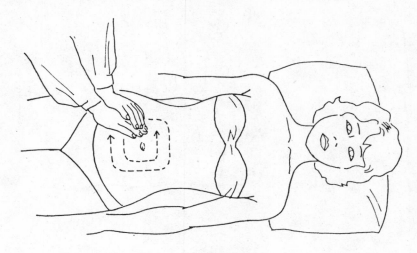

**Fig. 3**

36), 3 *cun* inferior to the lateral aspect of the knee and one finger's breadth lateral to the tibial crest, for one minute (fig. 4).

(5) Pinching along the spine

The patient lies prone with the back naked. The manipulator half clenches the fists with thumbs stretched out and the index and middle fingers propped on the coccygeal region, then pushing the right and left hand forward alternately along the Governor Vessel up to the seventh cervical vertebra while pinching (fig. 5). After three pushes and pinches, lift the skin upward and backward with force to enhance the stimulation of the acupoints related to visceral organs.

*2. Self-massage*

This is chiefly aimed at improving the constitution, and strengthening the tonus of the abdominal and gastric walls.

(1) Rubbing of the lumbo-sacral region

Take a sitting position. Place the palms closely against the lumbar region and rub it down to the sacral region (fig. 6). Repeat the manipulation for two minutes.

(2) Up-lifting of the sacrum and buttocks and at the same time contracting of the perineum

Lying supine with the legs bent and the soles of feet on the bed, lift up the sacrum and

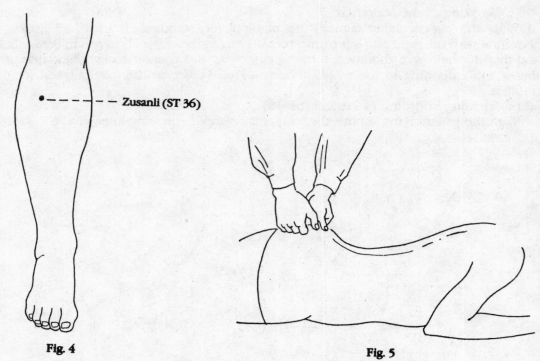

Zusanli (ST 36)

Fig. 4

Fig. 5

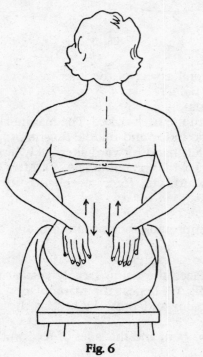

Fig. 6

buttocks as much as possible and at the same time contract the perineum, and then lie down flat (fig. 7). Repeat the movements again and again for about five minutes.

(3) Sit-ups

Lie supine with the legs stretched straight. Lift the head, chest and upper limbs when doing sit-ups and then lie down flat (fig. 8). Repeat the movements for 2-5 minutes.

NB:

(1) Perseveringly doing acupoint massage twice daily in the morning and in the evening will be effective for treating gastroptosis either of mild type or of severe type.

(2) It is recommended to have frequent, small meals. Eating and drinking too much at one meal and strenuous physical exercise after meals should be avoided, and appropriate alternation of work with rest and recreation is advised.

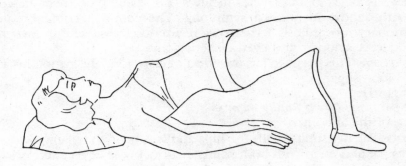

Fig. 7

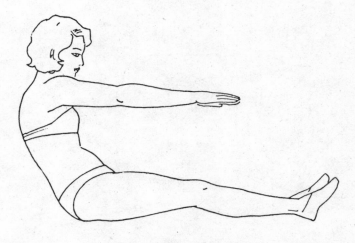

Fig. 8

# Diabetes Mellitus

Cause: Diabetes mellitus is a disease of unknown cause, characterized by chronic endocrine and metabolic disorders. Most scholars hold that this disease is chiefly due to decreased secretion of insulin or relatively increased insulin requirements of the body, either of which leads to metabolic disorders, especially disorders in glucose metabolism.

In traditional Chinese medicine, diabetes mellitus was recorded in the *Canon of Medicine*, a book compiled as early as the fourth century B.C. Its cause is there given as chiefly a constitutional deficiency of *yin* with overeating of fatty and sweet food or excessive drinking of alcoholic liquors, and emotional stress such as anxiety and anger.

Main Symptoms: Usually there are no symptoms at the early stage, and the disease is found by increased blood sugar level. A patient with diabetes mellitus of moderate severity may complain of excessive thirst, strong hunger, and a constant need to urinate, accompanied by fatiguability and loss of body weight. Glucose is present in the urine, and the blood sugar level is elevated. In diabetes mellitus of a severe type, there are complications in addition to the above-mentioned symptoms. The common complications are acute infection, pulmonary tuberculosis, hypertension, arteriosclerosis, and in a very severe case there may be ketosis, acidosis, and even diabetic coma.

Acupoint Massage: This massage has the effect of alleviating the symptoms and reducing the urine and blood sugar.

[Manipulation]

1. *Massage performed by a family member*

(1) Stroking of the abdomen

With the patient lying supine with the hips and legs bent, the manipulator, standing to the side, strokes the abdomen with both palms in a clockwise or counterclockwise circular movement around the umbilicus (fig. 1).

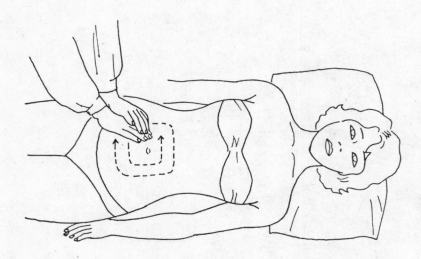

Fig. 1

(2) Point-pressing of Chengjiang (CV 24), Baihui (GV 20), Cuanzhu (BL 2) and Taiyang (EX-HN 5)

With the patient lying on the side, the manipulator, sitting behind, applies point-pressing with the tips of the thumbs or index fingers to Chengjiang (CV 24) at the midpoint of the mentolabial sulcus, Baihui (GV 20), 7 *cun* superior to the posterior hairline, at the midpoint of the line extending over the vertex joining the apexes of the auricles, Cuanzhu (BL 2) in the depression at the medial end of the eyebrow, and Taiyang (EX-HN 5) in the depression 1 *cun* superio-lateral to the external canthus (outer corner) of the eye, each for thirty seconds (fig. 2).

(3) Pushing of the face

With the patient lying supine, the manipulator, sitting behind, applies pushing to the patient's forehead with the ventral aspect of the thumbs longitudinally and horizontally for one minute, and then along the forehead, around the orbits and to the cheeks and mentolabial sulci with the hypothenar eminence for about two minutes (fig. 3).

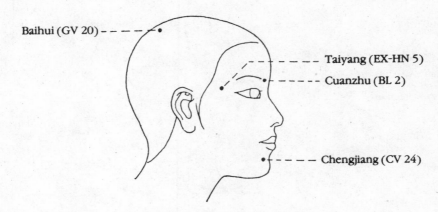

Baihui (GV 20)
Taiyang (EX-HN 5)
Cuanzhu (BL 2)
Chengjiang (CV 24)

**Fig. 2**

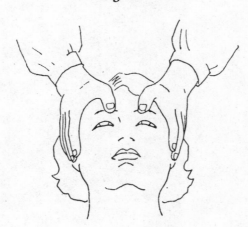

**Fig. 3**

(4) Pressing of Neiguan (PC 6), Hegu (LI 4), Zusanli (ST 36) and Sanyinjiao (SP 6)

With the patient lying supine, the manipulator applies pressing with the tip of thumbs to Neiguan (PC 6) on the anterior aspect of the forearm, 2 *cun* superior to the wrist crease, Hegu (LI 4) on the dorsum of the hand, between the first and second metacarpal bones on the radial aspect of the second metacarpal, Zusanli (ST 36), 3 *cun* inferior to the lateral aspect of the knee and one finger's breadth lateral to the tibial crest, and Sanyinjiao (SP 6) on the medial aspect of the leg, 3 *cun* superior to the tip of the medial malleolus, each for thirty seconds (fig. 4)

(5) Pressing-kneading of Bladder Meridian lateral to the spine

With the patient lying prone, the manipulator, standing to the side, pushes the palm forward (right and left palm alternately) while kneading the back along the Bladder Meridian lateral to the spine from the upper to the lower or vice versa (fig. 5). Repeat this for five minutes. Stress should put on the following points: Geshu (BL 17), 1.5 *cun* lateral

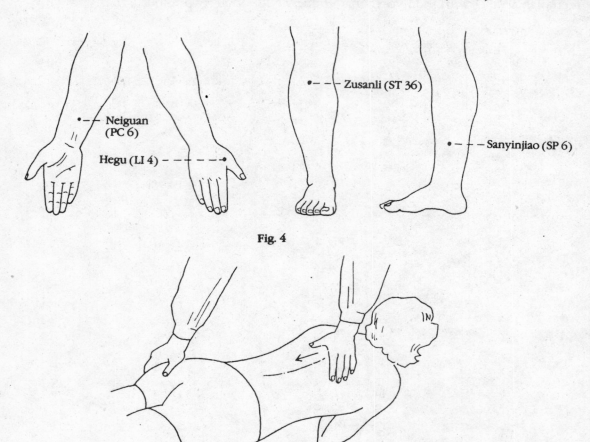

Neiguan (PC 6)

Hegu (LI 4)

Zusanli (ST 36)

Sanyinjiao (SP 6)

Fig. 4

Fig. 5

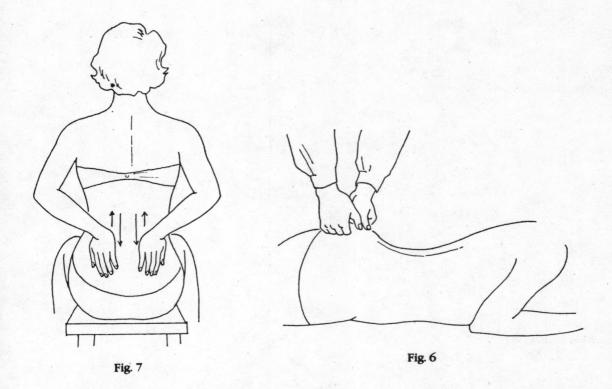

Fig. 7

Fig. 6

to the midpoint between the spinous processes of the seventh and eighth thoracic vertebrae; Ganshu (BL 18), 1.5 *cun* lateral to the midpoint between the spinous processes of the ninth and tenth thoracic vertebrae; Pishu (BL 20), 1.5 *cun* lateral to the midpoint between the spinous processes of the eleventh and twelfth thoracic vertebrae; and Shenshu (BL 23), 1.5 *cun* lateral to the midpoint between the spinous processes of the second the third lumbar vertebrae.

(6) Pinching along the spine

With the patient lying prone, the manipulator props the index and middle fingers of both hands on the coccyx and pushes the hands (the right and left hand alternately) forward along the Governor Vessel up to the seventh cervical vertebra while pinching (fig. 6). After three pushes and pinches, lift the skin once. Repeat the manipulation for 3-5 times.

2. *Self-massage*

(1) Rubbing of the lumbo-coccygeal region

Take a sitting position. Place the palms closely against the lumbar region and rub the skin down to the coccygeal region (fig. 7). Repeat this for one minute.

(2) Pushing of the abdomen

Lie supine. Place the palms on the lateral aspects of the abdomen and push the abdomen from the upper to the lower for about three minutes (fig. 8).

(3) Pressing-kneading of Laogong (PC 8) and Gongsun (SP 4)

Take a sitting position. Apply pressing-kneading with the tips of the thumbs to Laogong (PC 8) in the centre of the palm, and Gongsun (SP 4) on the medial aspect of the foot, in

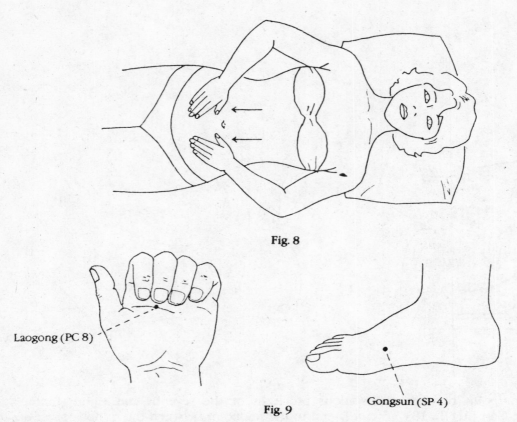

**Fig. 8**

Laogong (PC 8)

**Fig. 9**

Gongsun (SP 4)

the depression at the anterio-inferior border of the distal end of the first metatarsal each for one minute (fig. 9).

NB:

(1) Acupoint massage performed 1-2 times daily is effective for treating mild and moderate diabetes mellitus.

(2) Proper dietary regimen and physical exercise are recommended. Colds should be prevented.


## Hiccups

Cause: Hiccups are an ailment due to paroxysmal spasmodic contraction of the diaphragm. It is often caused by eating too fast or too much, sudden inhalation of cold air, stimulation of the intestines or emotional upsets. It also occurs in aged people of weak constitution, during a chronic or severe disease, after a surgical operation or during an attack of hysteria.

Main Symptoms: Repeated occurrence of sudden stopping of the breath along with a cough-like sound.

Acupoint Massage: This massage has the effect of relieving hiccups.

## [Manipulation]

### 1. Massage performed by a family member

(1) Stroking of the abdomen

With the patient lying supine with the legs bent, the manipulator, standing to the patient's right side, strokes the abdomen with both palms around the umbilicus, starting from the right lower abdomen and forming a clockwise circular movement (fig. 1). Repeat this for five minutes. The manipulation should be soft, gentle and appropriate in depth.

(2) Pressing-kneading of the back

With the patient lying prone, the manipulator, standing to the side, applies pressing-kneading with the right and left palm alternately to the back along the Bladder Meridian from the upper to the lower for three minutes (fig. 2).

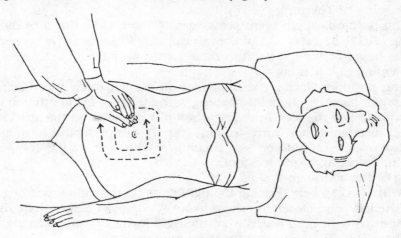

Fig. 1

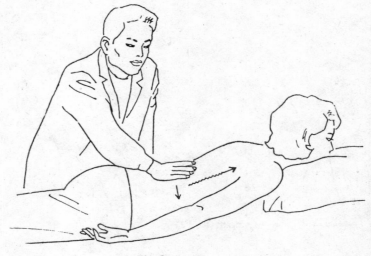

Fig. 2

(3) Point-pressing of Quepen (ST 12)

With the patient taking a sitting position, the manipulator, standing to the side, applies point-pressing with a thumb or middle finger to Quepen (ST 12) in the centre of supraclavicular fossa, 4 *cun* lateral to the anterior midline, for about thirty seconds (fig. 3). It is preferable to induce a feeling of numbness radiating to the chest.

(4) Point-pressing of Neiguan (PC 6)

The manipulator applies point-pressing with the tips of the thumbs to both Neiguan (PC 6) on the anterior aspect of the forearm, 2 *cun* superior to the wrist crease between the two tendons, for one minute (fig. 4). It is preferable to induce a feeling of soreness and distension.

*2. Self-massage*

(1) Point-pressing of Tianzong (SI 11)

Take a sitting position. Apply point-pressing with the middle finger of the right hand to left Tianzong (SI 11) in the centre of the infraspinous fossa for thirty seconds, and then with the middle finger of the left hand to right Tianzong (fig. 5).

(2) Point-pressing of Taichong (LR 3)

Take a sitting position. Placing the right foot on the left thigh and holding the right shank with the right hand, apply point-pressing with the tip of the left thumb to Taichong (LR 3) on the dorsum of the foot in the depression 2 *cun* distal to the articulation of the first and second metatarsals, for thirty seconds (fig. 6). It is preferable to induce a feeling of soreness, distension and numbness, radiating to the sole of the foot. Then apply point-pressing to Taichong of the left foot.

(3) Stroking of the abdomen

Lie supine with the legs bent. Placing the right palm on the right lower quadrant of the abdomen and the left palm closely on the dorsum of the right hand, stroke the abdomen around the umbilicus with both hands from the right lower upward, forming a clockwise circular movement (fig. 7). Repeat this for three minutes.

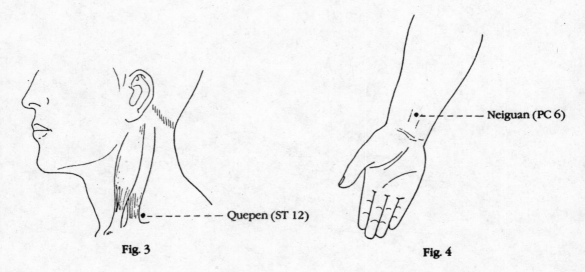

Fig. 3 — Quepen (ST 12)

Fig. 4 — Neiguan (PC 6)

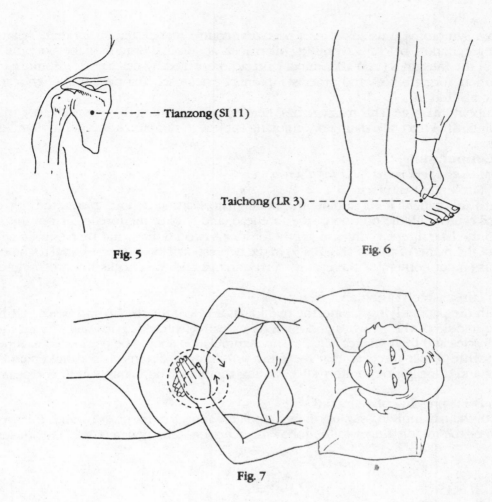

Tianzong (SI 11)

Taichong (LR 3)

Fig. 5

Fig. 6

Fig. 7

NB:

(1) Acupoint massage is effective for treating hiccups of non-organic origin. It should be done twice a day, in the morning and in the evening.

(2) Keeping a regular diet with avoidance of cold or spicy food is advised. Emotional upsets should be prevented.

## Gastrointestinal Neurosis

Cause: Gastrointestinal neurosis is a disease characterized by deranged secretory and motor functios of the gastrointestinal tract due to higher nervous functional disorders, although there is no organic lesion in the gastrointestinal tract itself. Its main causes are long-standing nervous tension, anxiety and improper diet, and sometimes it may be a sequela of colitis and dysentery.

Main Symptoms: It usually runs a persistent course, manifested by anorexia, heart-burn, acid regurgitation, belching, vomiting, diarrhoea, abdominal distension, borborygmi (rumbling in the intestines) and abdominal pain, accompanied by headaches, insomnia, cardiac palpitation, forgetfulness and other symptoms of neurosis. The patient is often lean with weak constitution.

Acupoint Massage: This massage has the effect of regulating the nervous function of the gastrointestinal tract, alleviating or removing subjective symptoms and improving digestive function.

**[Manipulation]**

*1. Massage performed by a family member*

(1) Stroking of the face

With the patient lying supine, the manipulator, sitting behind, places the tips of the thumbs on the middle portion of the forehead, and strokes the forehead from the medial part to the lateral repeatedly and gently for about two minutes; and then (stroke with the heels of the palms) Taiyang (EX-HN 5) in the depression 1 *cun* superio-lateral to the extenal canthus (outer corner) of the eye, its surroundings and the cheeks for two minutes (fig. 1).

(2) Lift-grasping of the abdomen

With the patient lying supine, the manipulator places the thumb and other four fingers on the middle of the patient's abdomen like a pair of pincers, grips and lifts up the skin and muscles and then relaxes (fig. 2). The manipulation should be performed in series and gently with proper force, so that there is a sensation of distension and mild pain during seizing and a feeling of comfort after loosing the hold. The manipulation is repeated 5-7 times.

(3) Point-pressing of acupoints

With the patient lying supine, the manipulator applies point-pressing with the tip of the thumb or the middle finger to the following acupoints: Zhongwan (CV 12), 4 *cun* superior

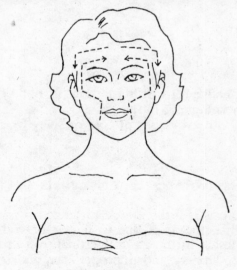

**Fig. 1**

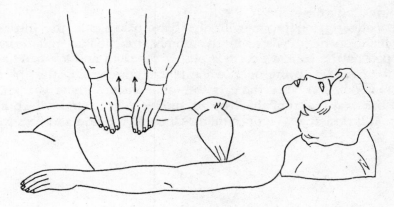

Fig. 2

to the umbilicus, Qihai (CV 6), 1.5 *cun* inferior to the umbilicus, Tianshu (ST 25), 2 *cun* lateral to the umbilicus, and Zusanli (ST 36), 3 *cun* inferior to the lateral aspect of the knee and one finger's breadth lateral to the tibial crest, each for thirty seconds with gradual increase of force (fig. 3). It is desirable to induce a feeling of mild soreness, distension, heaviness and numbness.

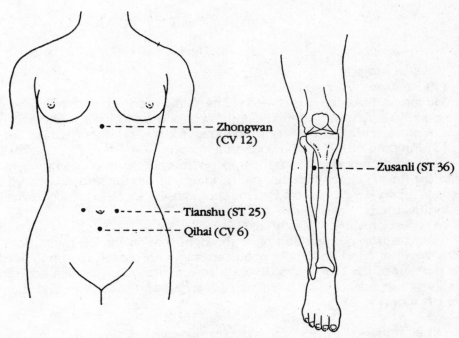

Fig. 3

(4) Pinching along the spine

With the patient lying prone with the back naked and the muscles relaxed, the manipulator half clenches the fists with the thumbs stretched out and the index and middle fingers propped on the patient's coccyx, pushes the right and left hand alternately along the Governor Vessel up to the neck while pinching, repeating this three times (fig. 4). During the manipulation, after three pushes and pinches, there is a lifting of the skin upward and backward accompanied by an audible "dla" sound, which indicates correct manipulation. It is desirable to induce mild redness of the skin and occasionally a burning sensation.

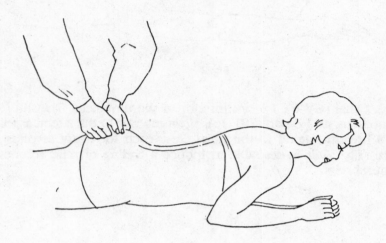

**Fig. 4**

*2. Self-massage*

(1) Stroking of the abdomen

Lie supine. Place the overlapped palms on the abdomen and stroke the abdomen around the umbilicus, first in the middle and lower portion in clockwise circular movements for five minutes, and then the whole abdomen for two minutes (fig. 5).

(2) Rubbing of the lumbo-coccygeal region

Take a sitting position with the upper portion of the trunk slightly bent. Place the palms with the fingers closed together on the loins and rub the skin downward to the coccygeal region (fig. 6). Repeat this for two minutes, causing slight redness of the skin with a feeling of local warmth.

(3) Point-pressing of Taichong (LR 3)

Take a sitting position and place the right foot on the left thigh. Hold the right shank with the right hand and apply point-pressing with the left thumb to Taichong (LR 3) on the dorsum of the foot, 2 *cun* distal to the articulation of the first and second metatarsals for thirty seconds, causing a feeling of soreness and distension, and then to Taichong of the left foot (fig. 7).

NB:

(1) It is advised to perform acupoint massage 1-2 times daily for 24 times, and then once every other day until the symptoms disappear.

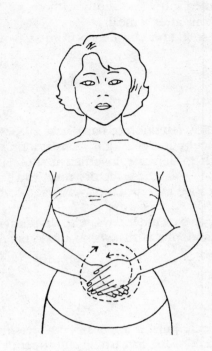

**Fig. 5**

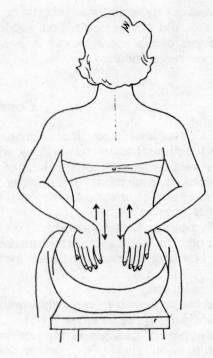

**Fig. 6**

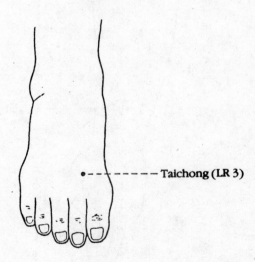

Taichong (LR 3)

**Fig. 7**

(2) Massage on the abdomen should be performed softly and gently without any violent actions. It should not be performed within one hour after a meal.

(3) Proper diet, a merry mood, a regular life style and abstinence from smoking and drinking are recommended.


# Constipation

Cause: Constipation is an ailment characterized by retention of hard fecal masses in the intestines for more than two days along with difficulty in defecation. Constipation may be caused by various factors, such as lack of strength to defecate, insufficient stimulation of the intestines, derangement of the nerve function — all these factors may lead to long-standing retention of intestinal contents with excessive absorption of water and formation of hard fecal masses.

Main Symptoms: Bowel movements once every two or more days, with dry fecal masses and difficulty in defecation, accompanied by abdominal distension, abdominal pain, dizziness, belching, anorexia and lassitude.
tion.

### [Manipulation]
*1. Massage performed by a family member*

(1) Point-pressing of Zhigou (TE 6)

With the patient taking a sitting position, the manipulator applies point-pressing with the thumb tips to Zhigou (TE 6) on the dorsal aspect of the forearm, 3 *cun* superior to the wrist crease between the radius and ulna, for thirty seconds (fig. 1).

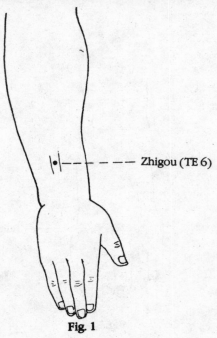

Zhigou (TE 6)

**Fig. 1**

68

(2) Point-pressing of Shangjuxu (ST 37)

With the patient lying supine, the manipulator applies point-pressing with the tip of the middle finger to Shangjuxu (ST 37), 6 *cun* inferior to the lateral aspect of the knee for thirty seconds (fig. 2).

(3) Pushing-kneading of the back

With the patient lying prone, the manipulator applies pushing while kneading with the palms to the back along the Bladder Meridian lateral to the spine from the lumbo-sacral region upward to the upper part of the back and then downward (fig. 3). Repeat the manipulation for three minutes.

(4) Rubbing of the lumbo-sacral portion

With the patient lying prone, the manipulator supports the waist with one hand, and rubs with the other palm the skin of the lumbo-sacral portion in a straight direction upward and downward or rightward and leftward with moderate pressure (fig. 4). The manipulation should be brisk with rapid movements, and mild redness of the skin with a feeling of warmth should be induced.

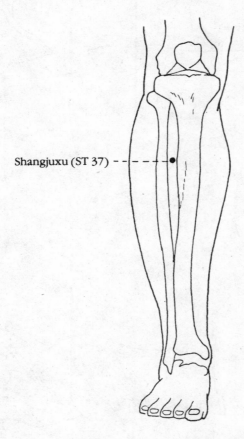

Shangjuxu (ST 37)

Fig. 2

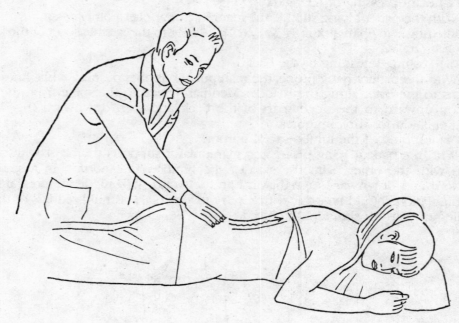

Fig. 3

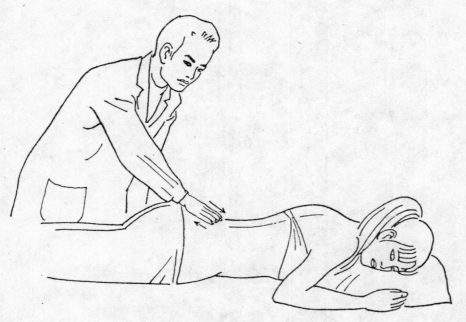

Fig. 4

## 2. Self-massage

(1) Stroking of the abdomen

Lie supine with the legs bent. Placing the palm of one hand on the back of the other hand, stroke the middle and lower portion of the abdomen around the umbilicus in clockwise circular movements for about five minutes and then the whole abdomen for two minutes (fig. 5). The manipulation should be brisk, soft and appropriate in depth, with the force light at first and then increased.

(2) Pushing-pressing of the left lower abdomen

Lie supine with the legs bent. Place the left palm on the left upper portion of the lower abdomen and the right palm on the back of the left hand. Push and press the abdomen with force from the upper to the lower with the two hands at the same time (fig. 6).

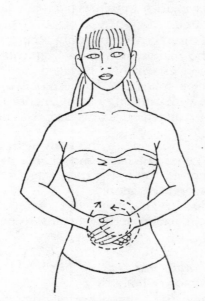

Fig. 5

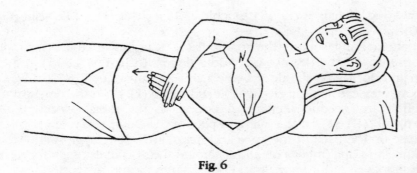

Fig. 6

NB:

(1) Acupoint massage performed daily in the morning and in the evening has good therapeutic and preventive effect for habitual and functional constipation.

(2) It is advised to make a habit of having bowel movements at a fixed time daily. Proper diet with adequate amount of vegetables and physical exercises are also of significance.

(3) Massage of the abdomen should be avoided within one hour before and after meals.

# Hemiplegia

Cause: In most cases hemiplegia is caused by cerebro-vascular accidents, but it can also occur in other brain diseases or injuries. In this section, only hemiplegia following cerebral thrombosis (blood clot) is discussed. When a blood clot obstructs a cerebral artery, hemiplegia is caused. Cerebral thrombosis commonly occurs in the middle cerebral artery, internal carotid artery and the middle and lower segments of basilar artery following arteriosclerosis and hypertension, especially in the aged.

Traditional Chinese medicine holds that the cerebral thrombosis is chiefly due to consumption of *qi* and blood with *yin-yang* derangement of the heart, liver, spleen and kidney with further impact of external affections, anxiety, anger, alcohol drinking, heavy meals or indulgence in sex.

Main Symptoms: Paralysis of one side of the body with a wry mouth and eye, stiff tongue and sluggish speech. The onset is often sudden, but may be gradual in some cases. The paralysis is spastic, although flaccid at the early stage; it may be accompanied by an entire or partial loss of motion and sensation.

Acupoint Massage: This massage has the effect of removing obstruction from the collaterals, promoting blood circulation and facilitating recovery of the functions of the limbs.

[Manipulation]

*1. Massage performed by a family member*

(1) Kneading the upper and lower limbs

With the patient lying supine, the manipulator, standing to the side, applies kneading with palms to the medial and lateral aspects of the upper and lower limbs from the upper to the lower for seven minutes, particularly to the shoulders, elbows, hips and knees (fig. 1).

(2) Point-pressing of Jianyu (LI 15), Quchi (LI 11), Hegu (LI 4), Fengshi (GB 31) and Zusanli (ST 36)

With the patient lying supine, the manipulator, standing to the side, applies point-pressing with the tips of the thumbs or middle fingers to Jianyu (LI 15) in the centre of the depression anterior to the shoulder as the arm is in full abduction, Quchi (LI 11) at the end of the elbow crease when the elbow is flexed, Hegu (LI 4) on the dorsum of the hand, between the first and second metacarpal bones, on the radial aspect of the second metacarpal, Fengshi (GB 31) on the lateral aspect of the thigh, 7 *cun* superior to the level of the skin crease on the back of the knee and Zusanli (ST 36), 3 *cun* inferior to the lateral aspect of the knee and one finger's breadth lateral to the tibial crest, each for thirty seconds (fig. 2). It is desirable to induce a feeling of local soreness and distension.

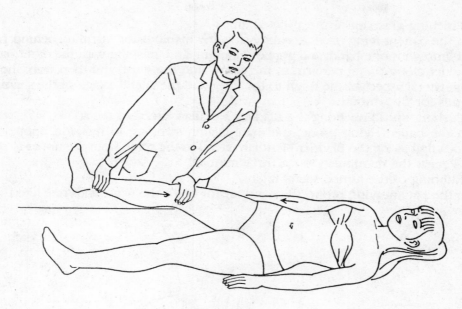

Fig. 1

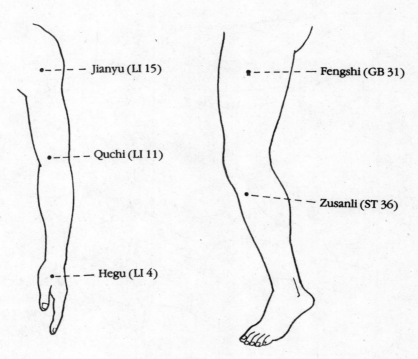

- — — — Jianyu (LI 15)

- — — — Fengshi (GB 31)

- — — — Quchi (LI 11)

- — — — Zusanli (ST 36)

- — — — Hegu (LI 4)

Fig. 2

(3) Pinching-grasping of the afflicted limbs

With the patient lying on the healthy side, the manipulator, standing behind, holds the afflicted limb with one hand, and applies pinching and grasping with the other hand from the shoulder along the upper arm to the elbow and the wrist, and then from the buttock along the lateral aspect of the thigh to the knee and the lateral aspect of the shank (fig. 3). Repeat this for five minutes.

(4) Pushing-kneading along the Bladder Meridian lateral to the spine

With the patient lying prone, the manipulator, standing to the side, applies pushing while kneading along the Bladder Meridian lateral to the spine from the upper to the lower (fig. 4). Repeat the manipulation for three minutes.

(5) Rubbing of the lumbo-sacral region

With the patient lying prone, the manipulator holds the waist with one hand, and rubs

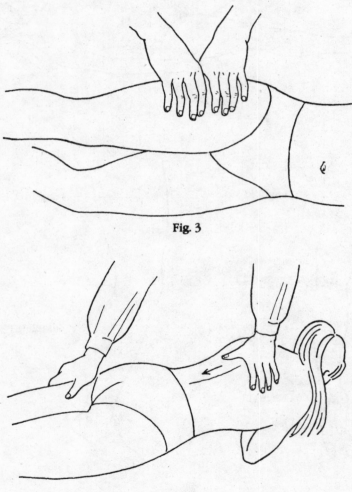

Fig. 3

Fig. 4

the skin with the palm of the other hand from the lumbar region to the sacral region for two minutes (fig. 5). It is desirable to induce a local feeling of warmth.

   2. *Self-massage*

   (1) Tapping of the afflicted limbs

   Take a sitting or supine lying position. Half clenching a fist with the healthy hand, tap the afflicted upper and lower limbs from the upper to the lower. Repeat this for 1-2 minutes.

   (2) Extending and flexing of the knee and ankle

   Take a sitting position. Lifting the leg with force, flex and then extend the knee and ankle joints. Repeat this for one minute.

   (3) Standing up and squatting down

   Stand with the support of a chair or the railing of a bed for one minute. Try to squat down with the support and then stand up (fig. 6). Repeat this for one minute.

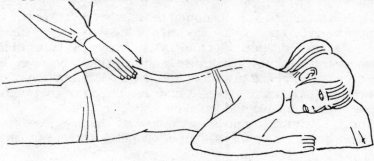

Fig. 5

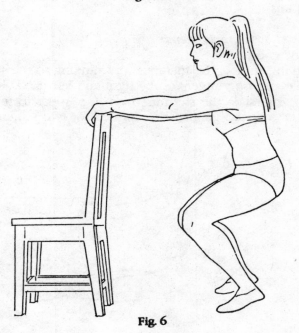

Fig. 6

NB:

(1) It is better to start acupoint massage two weeks after the onset of hemiplegia, performing it once daily or every other day with soft and gentle manipulation.

(2) During the massage, appropriate functional training should be started as soon as there is active movement of the afflicted limbs. As a rule, the active movement of the lower limb recovers earlier than that of the upper limb. In this case the patient is advised to stand and walk with a support and receive stimulation on the upper limb while sitting or standing.

(3) It is important to keep a merry mood and a regular lifestyle. Anxiety and anger should be avoided.

# Leukopenia

Cause: Leukopenia is defined as reduction in the number of leukocytes in the peripheral blood, the count being 4,000 per cubic millimetre or less, while the differential count may be normal or show slight reduction of granulocytes. Usually the patient has no complaints other than dizziness and weakness. The cause is not very clear; however, leukopenia often occurs in some bacterial, viral and protozoal infections, administration of certain drug and exposure to x-rays and radioactive agents. It may also be secondary to other diseases such as hypersplenism, aplastic anemia and leukemia.

Main Symptoms: Lassitude, dizziness, weakness of the legs, low fever, nausea and impaired sleep. The leukocyte count of the peripheral blood is less than 4,000 per cubic millimetre.

Acupoint Massage: This massage has the effect of increasing leukocyte count and improving the symptoms.

**[Manipulation]**

*1. Massage performed by a family member*

(1) Kneading of the chest

With the patient lying supine, the manipulator, standing to the side, applies kneading with the index, middle and ring fingers of the right and left hand alternately to the chest over the sternum and lateral to the sternum, from the upper to the lower (fig. 1). The manipulation should be soft and gentle, and repeated for two minutes.

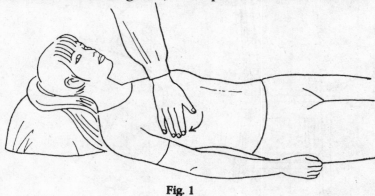

Fig. 1

(2) Pushing of the intercostal spaces

With the patient lying supine, the manipulator, standing behind and placing the palms with the fingers separate against the intercostal spaces, applies pushing from the sternum laterally to the armpits, and from the uppermost intercostal space to the lower spaces one by one (fig. 2). Repeat the manipulation for three minutes.

(3) Point-pressing of Xuehai (SP 10), Zusanli (ST 36) and Sanyinjiao (SP 6)

With the patient lying supine, the manipulator, standing to the side, applies point-pressing with the thumb tips to Xuehai (SP 10), 2 *cun* superior to the medial border of the patella, Zusanli (ST 36), 3 *cun* inferior to the lateral aspect of the knee and one finger's breadth lateral to the tibial crest, and Sanyinjiao (SP 6), 3 *cun* superior to the tip of the medial malleolus and just posterior to the tibia, each for one minute (fig. 3). It is desirable to induce a feeling of soreness and distension.

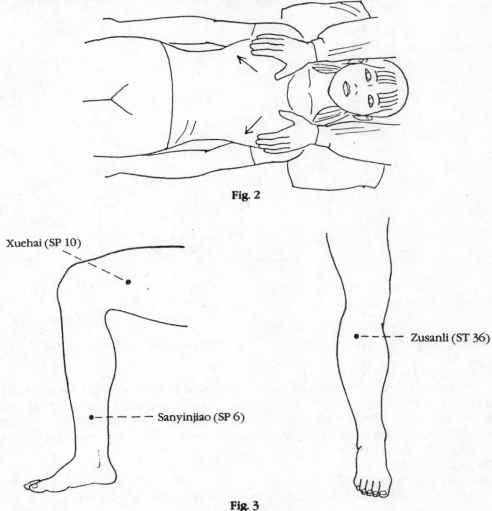

**Fig. 2**

Xuehai (SP 10)

Zusanli (ST 36)

Sanyinjiao (SP 6)

**Fig. 3**

(4) Stroking of the abdomen

With the patient lying supine with the hips and legs bent, the manipulator, standing to the side, strokes the abdomen with the right and left palm alternately around the umbilicus in clockwise circular movements for seven minutes (fig. 4). The manipulation should be brisk, soft and appropriate in depth.

(5) Pressing of Geshu (BL 17), Ganshu (BL 18), Pishu (BL 20) and Shenshu (BL 23)

With the patient taking a sitting position, the manipulator, sitting behind, applies point-pressing with the thumb tips to Geshu (BL 17), 1.5 *cun* lateral to the midpoint between the spinous processes of the seventh and eighth thoracic vertebrae, Ganshu (BL 18), 1.5 *cun* lateral to the midpoint between the spinous processes of the ninth and tenth thoracic vertebrae, Pishu (BL 20), 1.5 *cun* lateral to the midpoint between the spinous processes of the eleventh and twelfth thoracic vertebrae, and Shenshu (BL 23), 1.5 *cun*

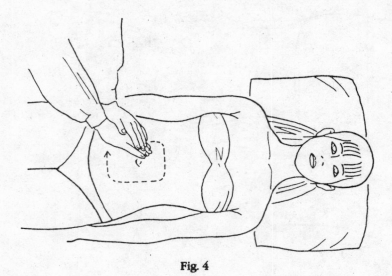

Fig. 4

lateral to the midpoint between the second and third lumbar vertebrae, each for one minute (fig. 5).

(6) Pinching along the spine

With the patient lying prone with the back naked and muscles relaxed, the manipulator props the index and middle fingers of both hands on the sacro-coccygeal region, pushes the right and left hand forward alternately while pinching along the Governor Vessel up to the seventh cervical vertebra, and lifts the skin upward after three pushes and pinches (fig. 6). Repeat the manipulation 3-5 times.

2. *Self-massage*

(1) Combing and rubbing of the head

Take a sitting position. Rub the scalp with the ten fingers slightly separate as with a comb (fig. 7). Repeat the manipulation for two minutes.

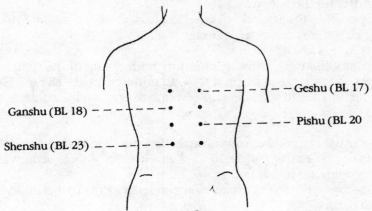

Geshu (BL 17)

Ganshu (BL 18)

Pishu (BL 20

Shenshu (BL 23)

**Fig. 5**

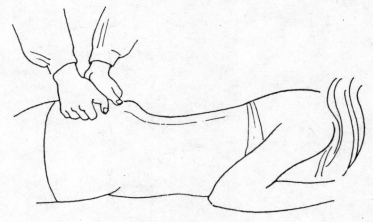

**Fig. 6**

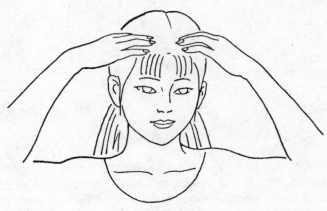

**Fig. 7**

(2) Rubbing of the lumbo-sacral region

Take a sitting position. Placing the palms closely against the skin of the lumbo-sacral region, repeatedly rubbing it for three minutes (fig. 8)

(3) Pressing-kneading of Diji (SP 8)

Take a sitting position. Apply pressing-kneading with the tip of the right and left middle finger to Diji (SP 8) of the same side, each for one minute (fig. 9). Diji (SP 8) is located on the posterior border of the tibia and 3 *cun* inferior to the medial condyle (ridge) of the tibia.

NB:

(1) Leukopenia usually runs a chronic course. It is recommended to perform acupoint massage daily or every other day for 20-40 days as a course of treatment, with a one-week interval before beginning a second course.

(2) Acupoint massage may have certain effect on leukopenia that is due to radiotherapy, chemotherapy and drugs.

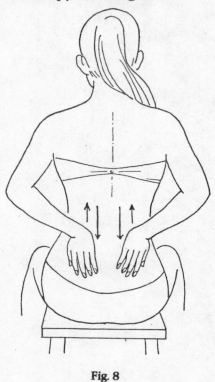

Fig. 8

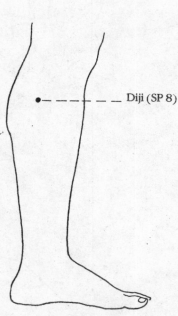

Diji (SP 8)

Fig. 9

## Neurasthenia

Cause: Neurasthenia, the most common variety of neurosis, is often caused by long-termed nervous tension, emotional upsets, persistent pondering, overfatigue or weakness after a disease, which leads to functional disorders of the cerebral cortex with resultant disturbances of autonomic nervous system and a series of symptoms.

According to traditional Chinese medicine, neurasthenia is often linked with insomnia and forgetfulness, mostly caused by emotional factors such as excessive joy, anger, melancholy, anxiety, grief, fear and terror, as well as overfatigue.

Main Symptoms: Insomnia, dream-disturbed sleep, restlessness, irritability, oversuspiciousness, headaches, dizziness, impaired memory, inability to concentrate, lassitute, weakness and listlessness; gastrointestinal symptoms such as nausea, belching, abdominal distension, anorexia and frequent bowel movements; menstrual disorders, impotence, premature ejaculation, seminal emission.

Acupoint Massage: This massage has the effect of regulating the balance between the excitory and inhibitory processes of the cerebral cortex, improving the autonomic nervous function and promoting health.

**[Manipulation]**

*1. Massage performed by a family member*

(1) Pushing of the forehead

With the patient lying supine, the manipulator, sitting behind, pushes the forehead both horizontally and longitudinally with the ventral aspect of the thumbs for two minutes (fig. 1).

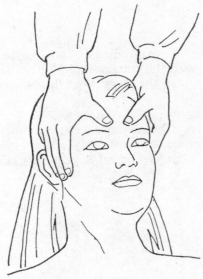

**Fig. 1**

(2) Pressing-kneading of Yintang (EX-HN 3), Taiyang (EX-HN 5), Neiguan (PC 6) and Zusanli (ST 36)

With the patient lying supine, the manipulator applies pressing-kneading with the tip of the thumb or middle finger to Yintang (EX-HN 3) at the midpoint between the eyebrows, Taiyang (EX-HN 5) in the depression 1 *cun* superio-lateral to the external canthus (outer corner) of the eye, Neiguan (PC 6) on the anterior aspect of the forearm, 2 *cun* directly superior to the midpoint of the wrist crease, and Zusanli (ST 36) 3 *cun* inferior to the lateral aspect of the knee and one finger's breadth lateral to the tibial crest, each for one minute (fig. 2).

81

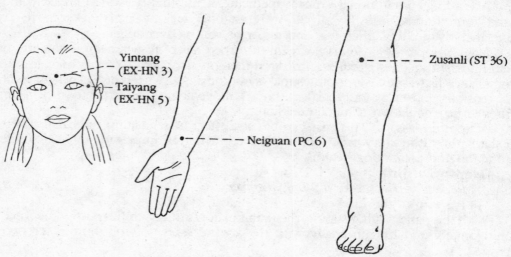

**Fig. 2**

(3) Pecking at the head

    With the patient lying supine, the manipulator, sitting behind, pecks at the head from the lateral aspects to the vertex with the fingers slightly bent and somewhat separate and with appropriate force exerting from the fingertips (fig. 3). Repeat the manipulation for two minutes.

(4) Stroking of the abdomen

    With the patient lying supine, the manipulator, standing to the side, strokes the abdomen with the right and left palm alternately around the umbilicus in clockwise movements from the medial to the lateral (fig. 4). Repeat the manipulation for five minutes.

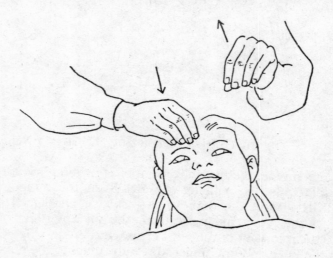

**Fig. 3**

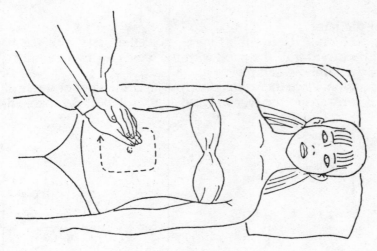

**Fig. 4**

(5) Pressing-kneading of the back along the Bladder Meridian lateral to the spine

With the patient lying prone, the manipulator, standing to the side, applies pressing while kneading with the right and left palm alternately to the back along the Bladder Meridian lateral to the spine from the seventh cervical vertebra to the lumbo-sacral region, particularly to Xinshu (BL 15), 1.5 *cun* lateral to the midpoint between the spinous processes of the fifth and sixth thoracic vertebrae, Shenshu (BL 23), 1.5 *cun* lateral to the midpoint between the spinous processes of the second and third lumbar vertebrae, and Mingmen (GV 4) in the depression between the spinous processes of the second and third lumbar vertebrae (fig. 5). Repeat the manipulation for five minutes.

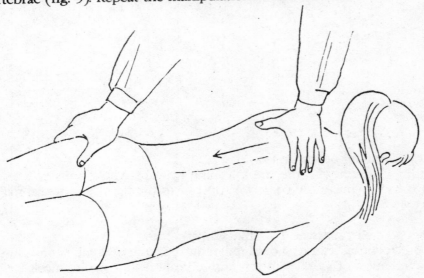

**Fig. 5**

*2. Self-massage*
(1) Rubbing of the nape
Take a sitting position. Crossing the fingers, hold the nape with the hands. Slightly bending the head backward, rub the nape with the hands for two minutes (fig. 6).
(2) Rubbing of the lumbo-sacral region
Take a sitting position. Place the palms closely against the sides of the small of the back, and rub the skin downward to the sacral region (fig. 7). Repeat the manipulation for two minutes.

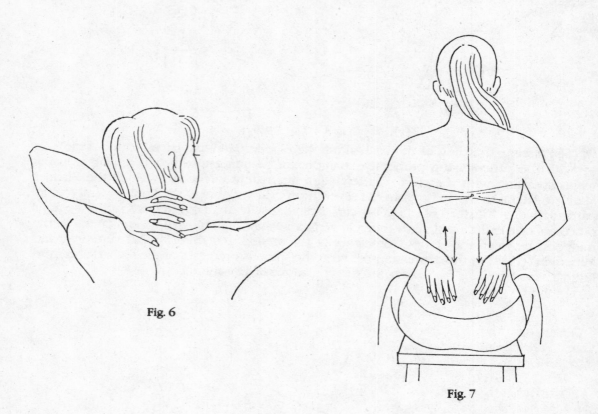

Fig. 6

Fig. 7

(3) Pressing-kneading of Sanyinjiao (SP 6)
Take a sitting position with the trunk leaning forward. Apply pressing-kneading with the thumb tips to Sanyinjiao (SP 6), 3 *cun* superior to the tip of the medial malleolus for two minutes (fig. 8).
NB:
(1) Perform acupoint massage 1-2 times daily.
(2) The precipitating cause should be removed, and mental stimulation avoided. Appropriate alternation of work with rest and recreation is of significance.
(3) Physical exercises, such as walking, leg-presses, squat-downs and stand-ups are recommended.

84

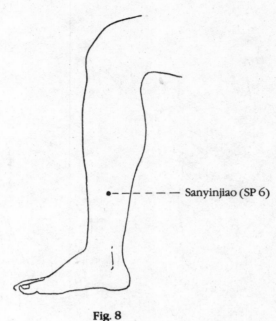

Fig. 8

# Insomnia

Cause: Insomnia is characterized by inability to sleep or abnormal wakefulness. There are a number of causes, among which anxiety, overfatigue, excessive nervous tension, interference from the surroundings, an irregular daily schedule and neurasthenia with nervous functional disorders are the common ones.

Traditional Chinese medicine holds that insomnia is due to disorders of the visceral organs and disharmony between *qi* and blood along with uneasiness of the mind.

Main Symptoms: Difficulty in falling asleep, abnormal wakefulness during sleep, dream-disturbed sleep, or even wakefulness all the night, often accompanied by dizziness, headaches, cardiac palpitation, indigestion, anorexia, tiredness and impairment of memory.

Acupoint Massage: This massage has the effect of causing sedation and inducing sleep.

[Manipulation]

*1. Massage performed by a family member*

(1) Stroking of the forehead and face

With the patient lying supine, the manipulator, sitting behind, places the ventral aspect of the thumbs on the middle portion of the forehead and repeatedly strokes the forehead from the medial to the lateral for three minutes (fig. 1), and then the parts lateral to the external canthus (outer corner) of the eye and the cheeks in clockwise circular movements for two minutes.

(2) Combing and causing vibration of the head

With the patient lying supine, the manipulator, sitting behind, rapidly combs the hair with slightly bent fingers from the anterior hairline to the temples and from the vertex to the occipitals, at the same time causing vibration of a frequency as high as possible (fig. 2). Repeat the manipulation for two minutes.

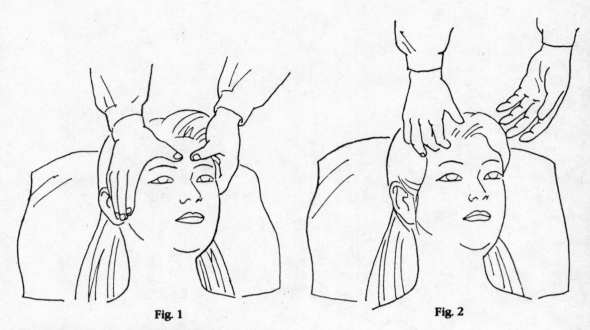

Fig. 1                                    Fig. 2

(3) Point-pressing of Shenmen (HT 7)

With the patient lying supine, the manipulator holds a wrist with one hand, and applies point-pressing with the thumb tip of the other hand to Shenmen (HT 7), just superior to the ulnar end of the ventral wrist crease, and then performs this on the other side, each for thirty seconds (fig. 3).

(4) Pressing-kneading of Sanyinjiao (SP 6)

With the patient lying supine, the manipulator applies pressing-kneading with the thumb tips to Sanyinjiao (SP 6), 3 *cun* superior to the tip of the medial malleolus, each for one minute (fig. 4)

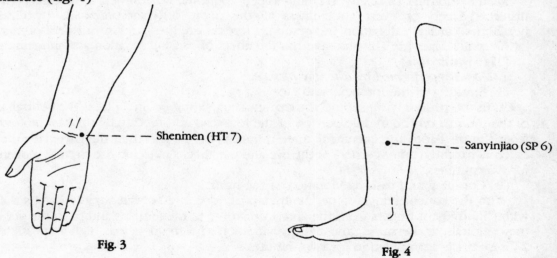

Shenmen (HT 7)                          Sanyinjiao (SP 6)

Fig. 3                                    Fig. 4

(5) Pushing-kneading of the back along the Bladder Meridian lateral to the spine

With the patient lying prone, the manipulator, standing to the side, applies pushing while kneading with the right and left palm alternately to the back along the Bladder Meridian lateral to the spine from the upper back to the lumbo-sacral region (fig. 5). Repeat the manipulation for five minutes.

*2. Self-massage*

(1) Squeezing-lifting of the nape

Take a sitting position. Crossing the fingers, hold the nape with the hands and slightly bend the head backward. Squeeze and lift and skin with the heels of the palms and then relax (fig. 6). Repeat the manipulation for one minute.

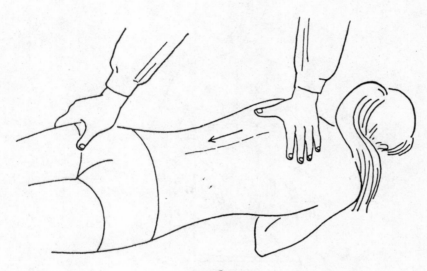

Fig. 5

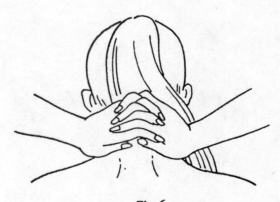

Fig. 6

(2) Rubbing of the lumbo-sacral region

Take a sitting position. Place the palms on the lumbo-sacral region closely against the skin and repeatedly rub the skin from the lumbar to the sacral regions for two minutes (fig. 7)

(3) Stroking of the abdomen

Lie supine with the legs bent. Overlapping the palms and placing them on the middle part of the abdomen, stroke the abdomen around the umbilicus in clockwise movements for three minutes (fig. 8). The manipulation should be soft with general relaxation and concentration of the mind on the lower abdomen.

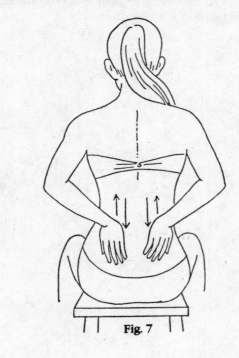

**Fig. 7**

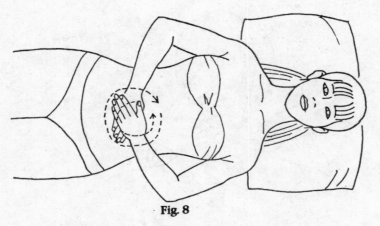

**Fig. 8**

NB:
(1) Perform the massage every evening before sleep.
(2) It is recommended to have a proper diet, regular daily schedule, appropriate alternation of work with rest and recreation and physical exercise.


# Hysteria

Cause: Hysteria often occurs in young women. It is a functional disease of the cerebral cortex, caused by various mental stimuli, emotional upsets or wicked suggestions. Generally, the patient is emotional, narrow-minded, sentimental, apt to be sulky, self-confident, imaginative, and suggestible.

According to traditional Chinese medicine, hysteria is a condition of mental disorder caused by violent emotions.

Main Symptoms: Various manifestations, including mental symptoms such as unreasonable crying, laughing, acting uproariously or dancing; motor disturbances such as aphasia, loss of voice, paralysis, tremors and spasms of the limbs; sensory disturbances such as sudden blindness, deafness or a sensation as if the throat is compressed; disorders of the visceral organs such as neurogenic vomiting or hiccups.

Acupoint Massage: This massage has the effect of calming the nerves and relieving the symptoms.

## [Manipulation]

(1) Nipping of Renzhong (also called Shuigou, GV 26)

With the patient lying supine, the manipulator, standing behind, presses hard with the tip of a thumb directly on Renzhong (GV 26), below the nasal septum at the upper one-third of the total length of the philtrum, alternating with relaxation rhythmically for about one minute until it causes a feeling of distension and pain (fig. 1).

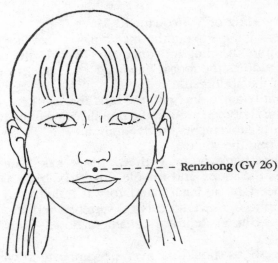

Renzhong (GV 26)

**Fig. 1**

(2) Point-pressing of Neiguan (PC 6), Hegu (LI 4) and Taichong (LR 3)

With the patient lying supine, the manipulator, standing to the side, applies point-pressing with the thumb tips to Neiguan (PC 6) on the anterior aspect of the forearm, 2 *cun* directly superior to the midpoint of the wrist crease between the two tendons, Hegu (LI 4) on the dorsum of the hand between the first and second metacarpal bones and on the radial aspect of the second metacarpal, and Taichong (LR 3) on the dorsum of the foot in the depression 1.5 *cun* distal to the articulation of the first and second metatarsals, each for one minute (fig. 2). It is desirable to induce soreness and distension.

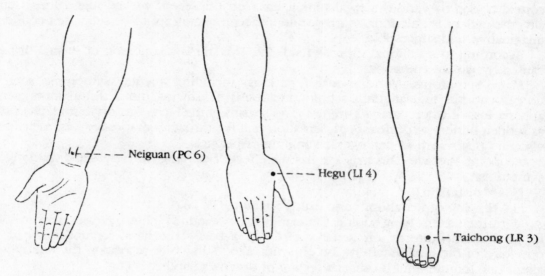

**Fig. 2**

(3) Pressing-kneading of Yongquan (KI 1)

With the patient lying supine, the manipulator, standing to the side, applies pressing and at the same time kneading to Yongquan (KI 1) in the centre of the sole of the foot and in the indentation as the foot is extended, each side for one minute (fig. 3).

(4) Stroking of the abdomen

With the patient lying supine with the hips and legs bent, the manipulator, standing to the side, strokes the abdomen around the umbilicus with the right and left palm alternately in clockwise circular movements for five minutes (fig. 4).

(5) Pinching along the spine

With the patient lying prone with the back naked and the muscles relaxed, the manipulator props the index and middle fingers of both hands on the sacro-coccygeal region, pushes the right and left hand forward alternately while pinching along the Governor Vessel up to the seventh cervical vertebra, and lifts up the skin once after three pushes and pinches (fig. 5). Repeat the manipulation 3-5 times.

NB:

(1) Verbal suggestions should be given in combination with massage.

(2) Keep the patient quiet and avoid any mental stimuli.

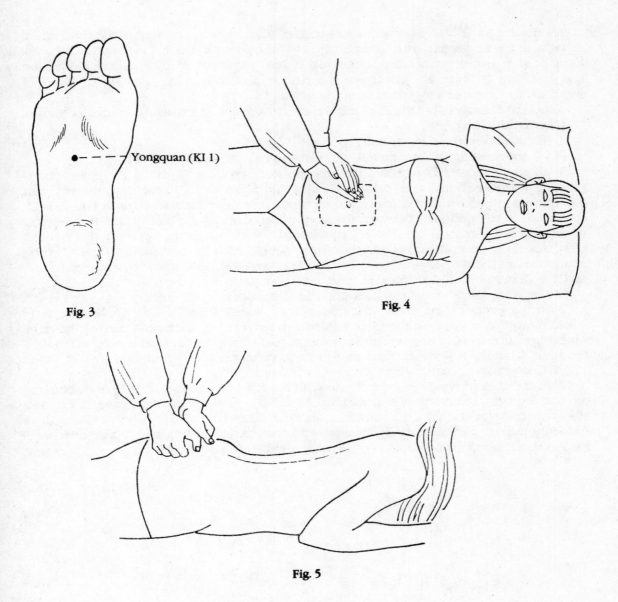

Fig. 3

Yongquan (KI 1)

Fig. 4

Fig. 5

## Biliary Colic

Cause: Biliary colic is a common symptom occurring in cholecystitis and cholelithiasis. Acupoint massage performed by a family member or the patient him or herself is chiefly used for the treatment of biliary colic in chronic cholecystitis. Biliary colic is usually produced by obstruction of the biliary tract with impaired bile excretion or spasm of the bile duct with acute expansion precipitated by taking greasy food or aggravation of the inflammation.

91

Main Symptoms: Dull pain with a sensation of distension and fullness in the epigastrium or right upper abdomen, usually occurring after a heavy meal or taking too much greasy food, or after nervous tension or emotional upsets, accompanied by anorexia, indigestion and belching. If there are gallstones, the pain is usually colicky, radiating to the right shoulder, accompanied by chills, fever, nausea and vomiting.

Acupoint Massage: This massage has the effect of relieving spasm and calming the pain.

**[Manipulation]**

*1. Massage performed by a family member*

(1) Point-pressing of Danshu (BL 19), Ganshu (BL 18) and Geshu (BL 17)

With the patient lying prone, the manipulator, standing to the side, applies point-pressing with the thumb tips to Danshu (BL 19), 1.5 *cun* lateral to the midpoint between the spinous processes of the tenth and eleventh thoracic vertebrae, Ganshu (BL 18), 1.5 *cun* lateral to the midpoint between the spinous processes of the ninth and tenth thoracic vertebrae, and Geshu ((BL 17), 1.5 *cun* lateral to the midpoint between the spinous processes of the seventh and eighth thoracic vertebrae, each for one minute (fig. 1). During manipulation, the thumb tip should be directed downward and to the thoracic vertebrae, and it is desirable to induce local soreness and distension.

(2) Pressing-kneading of the back and the right suprascapular region

With the patient lying prone, the manipulator, standing to the side, applies pressing-kneading to the back along the Bladder Meridian for seven minutes, and then to the right suprascapular region, giving strong stimulation particularly to the tender points lateral to the spine from the seventh to the tenth thoracic vertebrae for two minutes (fig. 2).

(3) Correction of the lower thoracic vertebral articulation

With the patient lying on the left side with the left leg stretched straight and the right hip and leg bent, the manipulator, standing to the side with the elbows flexed, places one elbow in front of the patient's shoulder and the other behind the patient's ilium, then suddenly pulls the patient's body forcibly with the elbows moving in opposite directions for 2-3 times, often accompanied by a clearly audible sound (fig. 3).

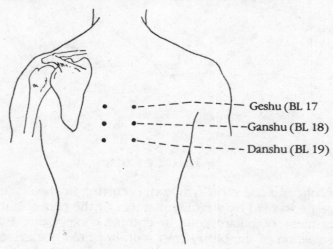

Geshu (BL 17
Ganshu (BL 18)
Danshu (BL 19)

**Fig. 1**

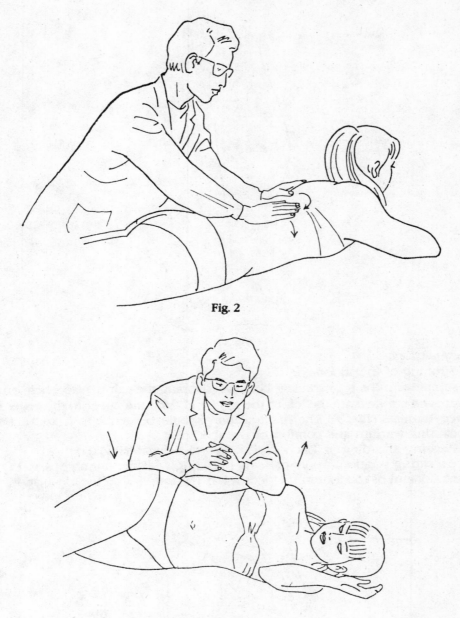

**Fig. 2**

**Fig. 3**

(4) Point-pressing of Yanglingquan (GB 34)

With the patient lying supine, the manipulator, standing to the side, applies point-pressing with the tip of overlapped thumbs to Yanglingquan (GB 34) in the depression anterio-inferior to the capitulum of the fibula, each side for one minute (fig. 4). Strong stimulation is preferred.

93

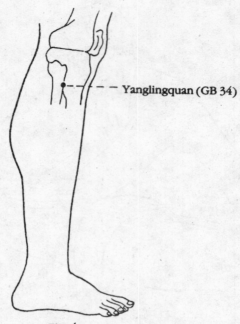

Fig. 4

## 2. Self-massage

(1) Stroking of the abdomen

Lie supine with the hips and legs bent. Overlapping the palms, place them on the upper abdomen, and stroke from the left to the right and from the upper to the lower repeatedly for seven minutes (fig. 5). The manipulation should be gentle, soft and appropriate in depth, causing warmth and comfort of the abdomen.

(2) Pressing-kneading of Taichong (LR 3) and Neiguan (PC 6)

Take a sitting position. Apply pressing-kneading with the thumb tips to Taichong (LR 3) on the dorsum of the foot in the depression 1.5 *cun* distal to the articulation of the first

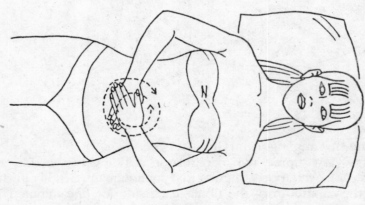

Fig. 5

and second metatarsals, and Neiguan (PC 6) on the anterior aspect of the forearm, 2 *cun* directly superior to the midpoint of the wrist crease, each for one minute (fig. 6).

NB:

(1) Acupoint massage performed daily or every other day can reduce or control the acute attacks of chronic cholecystitis and improve the symptoms.

(2) Too much drinking or eating at one meal and greasy food should be avoided. Keep a merry mood and have appropriate alternation of work with rest and recreation.

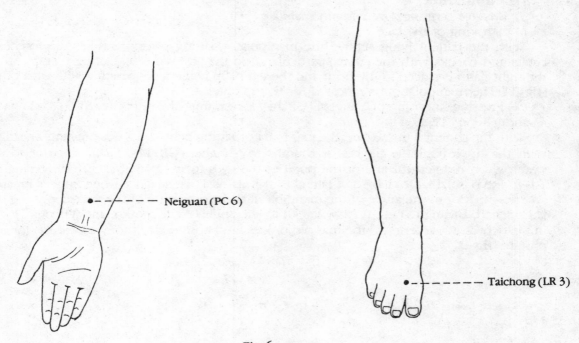

Neiguan (PC 6)

Taichong (LR 3)

Fig. 6

## Facial Paralysis

Cause: Peripheral facial paralysis is a syndrome of acute nonsuppurative inflammation of the facial nerve in the stylomastoid foramen, which may be due to ischemia and edema of the nerve consequent upon the spasm of its blood vessels after exposure to wind and cold, or due to a local virus infection. In addition, facial paralysis may also be secondary to chronic otitis media and mastoiditis.

Traditional Chinese medicine holds that this disease is caused by the attack of the face by wind and cold which leads to stagnation in the meridians and collaterals and consequently deranged nutrition of the nerve when the human body is in deficiency of *qi* and blood.

Main Symptoms: In some cases, there is a discomfort feeling of the affected side of the face before the onset of paralysis. In most cases, impairment of eye closure and retraction of the angle of the mouth is accidentally found in the morning on waking up, followed by aching pain about the angle of the jaw or behind the ear, loss of facial expression, inability to close the eye and frown, deviation of the mouth angle to the healthy side, shallowing of the nasolabial sulcus, indistinct speech, difficulty in pushing out of the cheek of the affected side. Taste perception on the anterior two thirds of the involved half of the tongue may be distorted or lost.

Acupoint Massage: This massage has the effect of improving the affected blood circulation and promoting the recovery of the nervous function.

**[Manipulation]**

*1. Massage performed by a family member*

(1) Stroking of the face

With the patient lying supine, the manipulator, sitting behind, strokes the forehead, orbits and cheeks with the palms, particularly on the affected side. During manipulation, the right palm is placed in the front and the left palm behind, cooperating with each other (fig. 1). The manipulation is repeated for five minutes.

(2) Pressing-kneading of Yangbai (GB 14), Yingxiang (LI 20), Jiache (ST 6), Dicang (ST 4) and Yifeng (TE 17)

With the patient lying supine, the manipulator, sitting behind, applies pressing-kneading with the tips of middle fingers or thumbs to Yangbai (GB 14), 1 *cun* superior to the eyebrow on the vertical line of the pupil as the eyes focus straight ahead, Yingxiang (LI 20) in the nasolabial fold, 0.5 *cun* lateral to the ala nasi, Jiache (ST 6), one finger's breadth anterio-superior to the angle of the mandible at the prominence of the masseter as the jaw is clenched, Dicang (ST 4), 0.4 *cun* lateral to the angle of the mouth, and Yifeng (TE 17) in the depression anterior to the mastoid process and posterior to the earlobe, each for one minute (fig. 2).

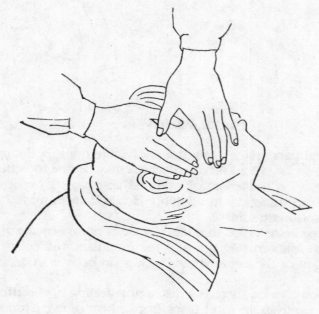

**Fig. 1**

96

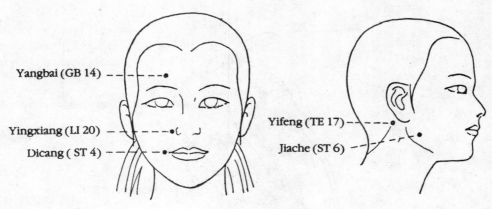

Yangbai (GB 14)

Yingxiang (LI 20)

Dicang ( ST 4)

Yifeng (TE 17)

Jiache (ST 6)

**Fig. 2**

(3) Pinching of the cheeks

With the patient lying supine, the manipulator, standing to the side with the hands half clenched in fists and the index fingers propped on the the angles of mandibles, gently pinches and lifts up the affected cheek with the thumb, index and middle fingers and then relaxes (fig. 3). The manipulation is repeated from the lower to the upper for one minute.

(4) Pressing-grasping of Fengchi (GB 20) and the neck and shoulder

The patient takes a sitting position. The manipulator, standing behind, supports the patient's forehead with one hand, and applies pressing and at the same time grasping with the thumb, index and middle fingers of the other hand to Fengchi (GB 20) at the base of the skull, in the depression between the heads of the sternocleidomastoid and trapezius muscles for two minutes, and then repeats the manipulation along the posterior and lateral aspects of the neck to the shoulder for three minutes (fig. 4).

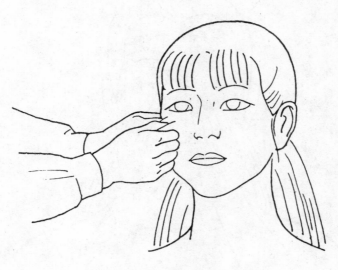

**Fig. 3**

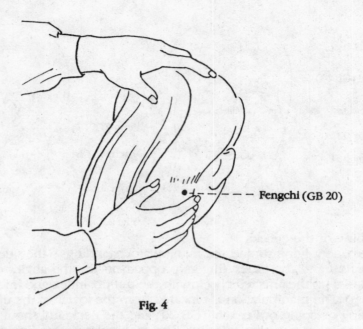

Fengchi (GB 20)

Fig. 4

## 2. Self-massage
(1) Pushing and stroking of the face

Take a sitting position. Rubbing the palms warm and placing them on the face, push and stroke the face from the mandible through the perioral region, cheeks, nasolabial sulci to the forehead (fig. 5). Repeat the manipulation for three minutes.

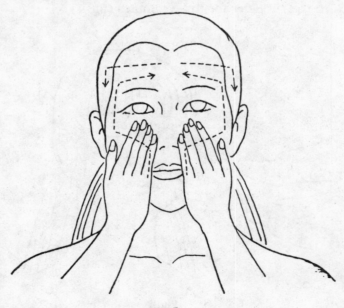

Fig. 5

(2) Kneading of the extra-ocular region and cheek

Take a sitting position. Place both hypothenars on the regions lateral to the eyes and cheeks and repeatedly knead the skin, particularly of the affected side for two minutes (fig. 6).

(3) Pushing out of the cheeks and pouting of the lips

Hold the affected half of the lips with the index and middle fingers of one hand, and push out the cheeks and pout the lips with effort to blow the air out through the healthy side. Perform the exercise three times a day, and in each exercise make 20 blows.

(4) Pressing-kneading of Hegu (LI 4) and Lieque (LU 7)

Take a sitting position. Apply pressing-kneading to Hegu (LI 4) on the dorsum of the hand between the first and second metacarpal bones and on the radial aspect of the second metacarpal, and Lieque (LU 7), 1.5 *cun* proximal to the wrist crease, immediately superior to the styloid process of the radius, each for one minute (fig. 7).

NB:

(1) Perform the acupoint massage twice a day, in the morning and in the evening. The manipulation should be soft and gentle with moderate force.

(2) Fatigue and local exposure to wind and cold should be avoided.

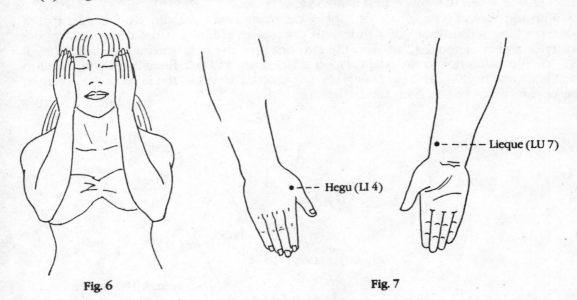

Fig. 6                                                        Fig. 7

## Raynaud's Disease

Cause: Raynaud's disease characterized by paroxysmal spasms of the digital arteries, is of unknown etiology. It often occurs in women. Some hold that it is due to central nervous derangement with abnormal sympathetic activity that leads to local ischemia, while others relate this disease with endocrine disturbances. The attack is often precipitated by cold and emotional stimuli.

Main Symptoms: The onset is usually gradual with attacks only in the winter after exposure to cold, especially exposure of the fingers to cold water. During the attack, the fingers of both hands blanch symmetrically, followed by cyanosis. The digits are cold and numb. During recovery, a bright red colour replaces the cyanosis and there is a burning, tingling sensation. In individual cases, there are skin atrophy and changes of the nails.

Acupoint Massage: This massage has the effect of regulating the autonomic nervous function, and alleviating or relieving peripheral vascular spasm.

[Manipulation]

*1. Massage performed by a family member*

(1) Point-pressing of Hegu (LI 4), Neiguan (PC 6) and Quchi (LI 11) of the affected side when the upper limb is involved

With the patient taking a sitting position, the manipulator applies point-pressing with the tip of a thumb to Hegu (LI 4) on the dorsum of the hand between the first and second metacarpal bones and on the radial aspect of the second metacarpal, Neiguan (PC 6) on the anterior aspect of the forearm, 2 *cun* superior to the midpoint of the wrist crease between the two tendons, and Quchi (LI 11) in the depression at the lateral end of the elbow crease as the elbow is flexed, each for one minute (fig. 1). It is desirable to induce a feeling of local soreness and distension.

(2) Point-pressing of Chengshan (BL 57), Zusanli (ST 36) and Weizhong (BL 40) of the affected side when the lower limb is involved

With the patient lying prone or supine, the manipulator, standing to the side, applies point-pressing with the tip of a thumb to Chengshan (BL 57) in the depression on the posterior aspect of the leg, between the two heads of the gastrocnemius muscle, Zusanli (ST 36), 3 *cun* inferior to the lateral aspect of the knee and one finger's breadth lateral to the tibial crest, and Weizhong (BL 40) on the posterior aspect of the knee, at the centre of the popliteal skin crease, each for one minute (fig. 2).

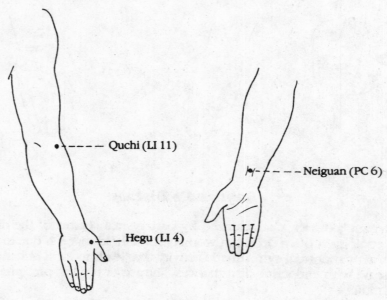

Quchi (LI 11)

Neiguan (PC 6)

Hegu (LI 4)

**Fig. 1**

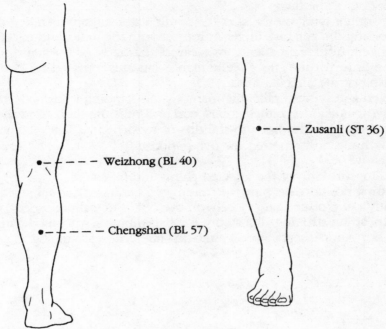

Weizhong (BL 40)

Chengshan (BL 57)

Zusanli (ST 36)

Fig. 2

### (3) Pinching-grasping of the affected limb

With the patient lying supine, the manipulator, standing to the side, using the thumb and other three fingers (index, middle and ring fingers) like a pair of pincers, applies pinching-grasping and relaxing alternately to the tendons and muscles of the affected limb from the elbow to the fingertips or from the knee to the tips of toes, and also from the lateral aspect to the medial (fig. 3). The manipulation is repeated for three minutes and the force used is as strong as the patient can tolerate.

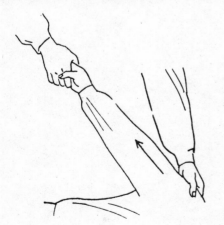
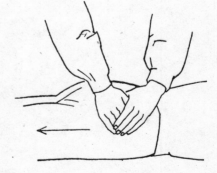

Fig. 3

(4) Squeezing of the digits

With the patient lying on the side, the manipulator, slightly bending the fingers of one hand and holding the patient's finger or toe between the index and middle fingers, rapidly slides the fingers from the patient's metacarpophalangeal or metatarsophalangeal joint to the tip of the finger or toe (fig. 4). The manipulation is repeated for one minute.

(5) Rubbing of the affected limb

With the patient lying supine, the manipulator, standing to the side, holds the affected limb with two palms on symmetrical aspects and rubs the limb from the shoulder to the tips of fingers or from the knee to the tips of toes (fig. 5). The manipulation should be brisk and rhythmic, and repeated for five minutes.

*2. Self-massage*

(1) Kneading-stroking of the affected palms and fingers

Take a sitting position. Keeping the thumb of a hand in a natural position and the other fingers slightly bent, place them closely on the dorsal or palmar aspect of the other hand and apply kneading-stroking repeatedly for five minutes with moderate and even force deep to the skin and subcutaneous tissue, causing local warmth (fig. 6).

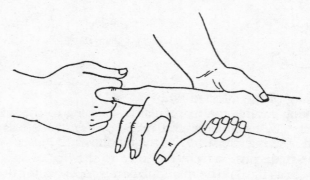

Fig. 4

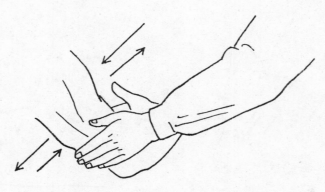

Fig. 5

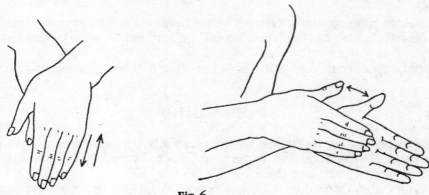

Fig. 6

(2) Twisting of the affected finger or toe

Take a sitting position, twist while pulling the affected finger or toe with the ventral aspect of the thumb, index and middle fingers rightward and leftward symmetrically, working from the metacarpophalangeal or metatarsophalangeal joint to the tip of the finger or toe (fig. 7).

(3) Stroking of the abdomen

Lie supine with the hips and legs bent. Overlapping the palms, place them on the abdomen closely against the skin, and stroke the abdomen around the umbilicus from the right to the left in circular movements (fig. 8). Repeat this for five minutes.

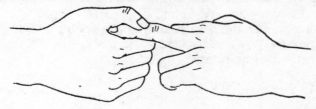

Fig. 7

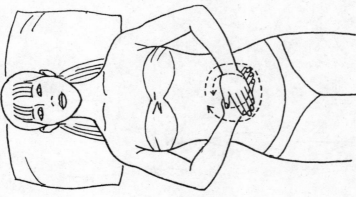

Fig. 8

NB:

(1) Acupoint massage once a day or in cold seasons 2-3 times a day may alleviate and prevent the attack. The manipulation should be soft, gentle with proper force to prevent abrasion.

(2) Avoid exposure to cold water in wintertime and keep the affected limbs warm.

## Prostatitis

Cause: Prostatitis may be caused by long-standing congestion of the perineum with a reduction in local resistance and bacterial infection, spread of urethritis to the prostate, indulgence in sex or excessive drinking.

Main Symptoms: Difficulty in urination with drippling of urine, dripping of whitish secretion at the end of urination, pain, urgency and frequency of urination, distension and pain in the lumbo-sacral region and perineum, sexual debility, seminal emission and premature ejaculation, accompanied by insomnia, lack of strength and dizziness.

Acupoint Massage: This massage has the effect of promoting blood circulation, lessening inflammation, reducing nervous tension and alleviating symptoms.

[Manipulation]

*1. Massage performed by a family member*

(1) Kneading of the lower abdomen

With the patient lying supine with the hips and legs bent, the manipulator, standing to the side, kneads the lower abdomen with two palms for five minutes (fig 1).

(2) Point-pressing of Guanyuan (CV 4) and Zhongji (CV 3)

With the patient lying supine, the manipulator applies point-pressing with the tip of the middle finger to Guanyuan (CV 4), 3 *cun* below the umbilicus, and Zhongji (CV 3), 4 *cun* below the umbilicus, each for one minute (fig. 2).

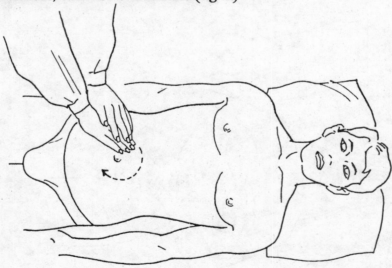

Fig. 1

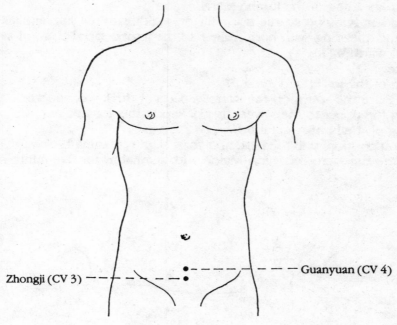

Zhongji (CV 3) - - - - - - - - - - - - - - - Guanyuan (CV 4)

**Fig. 2**

(3) Pressing-kneading of Yinlingquan (SP 9) and Sanyinjiao (SP 6)

With the patient lying supine, the manipulator applies pressing-kneading with the thumb tips to Yinlingquan (SP 9) in the depression on the medial aspect of the knee, inferior to the medial condyle of the tibia, and Sanyinjiao (SP 6), 3 *cun* superior to the tip of the medial malleolus and just posterior to the tibia, each for one minute (fig. 3).

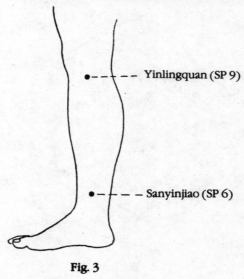

Yinlingquan (SP 9)

Sanyinjiao (SP 6)

**Fig. 3**

(4) Pushing-kneading of the lumbo-sacral region

With the patient lying prone, the manipulator, standing to the side, applies pushing and at the same time kneading with both palms to the lumbo-sacral region for five minutes to induce local warmth (fig. 4).

*2. Self-massage*

(1) Pushing of the lower abdomen

Lie supine. Place the palms on the lateral aspects of the lower abdomen, and push the abdomen from the upper to the lower (fig. 5). Repeat this for five minutes.

(2) Rubbing of the lumbo-sacral region

Take a sitting position with the head and chest slightly leaning backward. Rub the loins from the waist to the sacro-coccygeal region with the palms for five minutes (fig. 6).

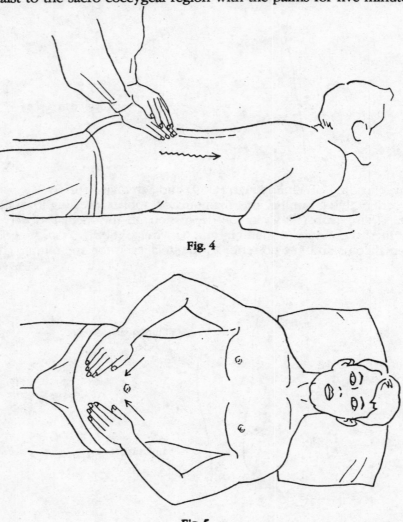

Fig. 4

Fig. 5

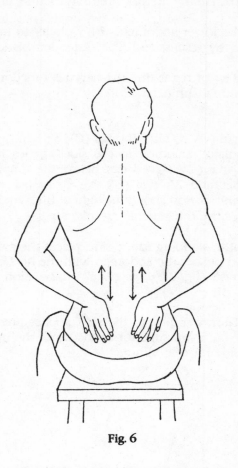

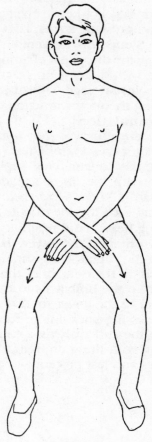

Fig. 6                                              Fig. 7

(3) Pinching of the medial aspect of the thigh

Take a sitting position. Pinch the medial aspect of the right thigh with the left hand and the medial aspect of the left thigh with the right hand from the groin to the knee (fig. 7). Repeat the manipulation for two minutes.

NB:

(1) Perform the massage twice daily, in the morning and in the evening. Restrain from sexual intercourse, keep the genitals clean and prevent urinary infection.

(2) Take a hot bath 1-2 times daily, each time for 15-25 minutes. The water temperature should be as high as the patient can tolerate.


## Retention of Urine

Cause: Retention of urine refers to accumulation of a large amount of urine in the bladder which can not be discharged voluntarily or is passed with difficulty. Its common causes are: nervous tension, neurological diseases, nerve injuries, spasm of the sphincter after abdominal or pelvic operations or due to pain in the urethra, urethral stricture, urinary stone and prostatic hyperplasia.

Main Symptoms: Intolerable distension of the lower abdomen with inability to urinate or only with drippling of urine, accompanied by restlessness. The distended bladder is palpable with dullness on percussion.

Acupoint Massage: This massage has the effect of regulating the nervous function and improving the motor function of the vesicourethral sphincter.

[Manipulation]

*1. Massage performed by a family member*

(1) Point-pressing of Qihai (CV 6), Guanyuan (CV 4) and Zhongji (CV 3)

With the patient lying supine, the manipulator, standing to the side, applies point-pressing with the tip of a middle finger to Qihai (CV 6), 1.5 *cun* below the umbilicus, Guanyuan (CV 4), 3 *cun* below the umbilicus, and Zhongji (CV 3), 4 *cun* below the umbilicus, each for one minute (fig. 1). The manipulation should be light at first, gradually becoming heavy until reaching the highest pressure the patient can tolerate.

(2) Pushing of the lower abdomen

With the patient lying supine, the manipulator, standing to the side, places the palm of one hand on the dorsum of the other hand and pushes the abdomen with the heel of the palms from the umbilicus to the pubic symphysis (fig. 2). Repeat the manipulation from the upper to the lower for five minutes.

(3) Pressing-kneading of Sanyinjiao (SP 6)

With the patient lying supine, the manipulator, standing to the side, applies pressing-kneading with the thumb tip to Sanyinjiao (SP 6), 3 *cun* superior to the tip of the medial malleolus and just posterior to the tibia, each side for one minute.

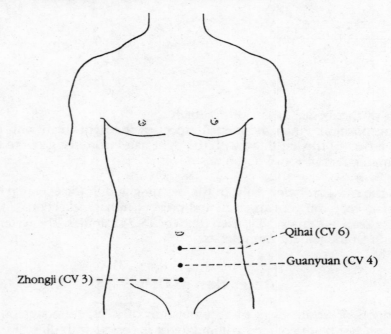

**Fig. 1**

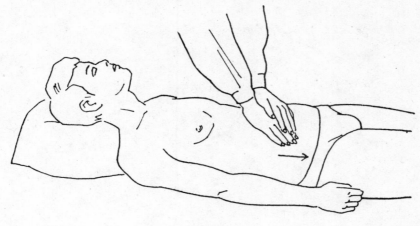

**Fig. 2**

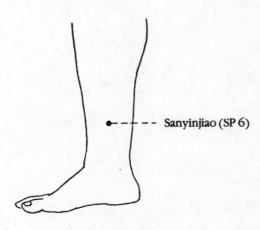

Sanyinjiao (SP 6)

**Fig. 3**

(4) Kneading of Pishu (BL 20) and Shenshu(BL 23)

With the patient lying supine, the manipulator, standing to the side, applies kneading with the ventral aspect of the thumbs to Pishu (BL 20), 1.5 *cun* lateral to the midpoint between the eleventh and twelfth thoracic vertebrae, and Shenshu (BL 23), 1.5 *cun* lateral to the midpoint between the second and third lumbar vertebrae, each for one minute (fig. 4).

(5) Rubbing of the lumbo-sacral region

With the patient lying prone, the manipulator, standing to the side, repeatedly rubs the lumbo-sacral region with the right and left palm alternately from the loins to the sacrum for two minutes to induce local warmth (fig. 5).

*2 Self-massage*

(1) Stroking of the lower abdomen

Lie supine with the hips and legs bent. Place the right palm on the lower abdomen and

109

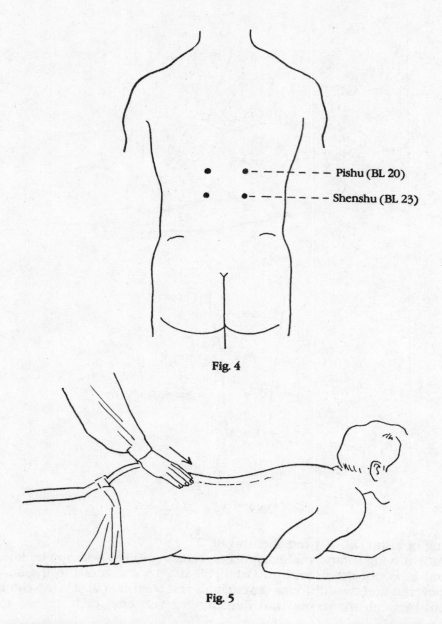

Pishu (BL 20)

Shenshu (BL 23)

Fig. 4

Fig. 5

the left palm on the dorsum of the right hand, and stroke the lower abdomen in circular movements, taking the midpoint between the umbilicus and the pubic symphysis as the centre (fig. 6). Repeat the manipulation for five minutes.

(2) Stirring of Yinlingquan (SP 9)

Take a sitting position. Stir the local tissue with the thumb tips at Yinlingquan (SP 9) in the depression on the medial aspect of the knee, inferior to the medial condyle of the tibia for one minute (fig. 7)

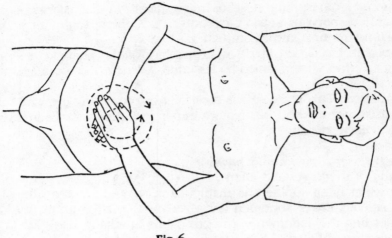

Fig. 6

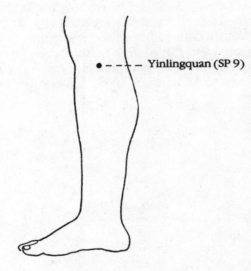

Yinlingquan (SP 9)

Fig. 7

NB:
(1) Acupoint massage should be performed 2-4 times a day.
(2) The manipulation should be even and soft with appropriate force.

## Impotence

Cause: Impotence refers to inability of the penis to erect or insufficient rigidity during erection. Only in the minority of cases impotence is caused by organic lesions of the reproductive organs such as anomaly, chronic inflammation (particularly chronic prostati-

111

tis), maldevelopment of testis and nervous injuries, while in the majority of cases impotence is functional, due to nervous tension, excessive excitement, fright, anger, anxiety, indulgence in sexual intercourse and masturbation.

Main Symptoms: Decreased libido with inability of the penis to erect or insufficient rigidity during erection, accompanied by lassitude, soreness and weakness of the loins and knees, and dizziness.

Acupoint Massage: This massage has the effect of promoting the vital functions and is therefore a satisfactory method for treating impotence. Perseverance in acupoint massage usually gives excellent results.

[**Manipulation**]

*1. Massage performed by a family member*

(1) Kneading of the lower abdomen

With the patient lying supine, the manipulator, standing to the side, places the right palm on the patient's lower abdomen and overlaps the left palm on the dorsum of the right hand, kneading the abdomen with both palms simultaneously (fig. 1).

(2) Point-pressing of Qihai (CV 6) and Guanyuan (CV 4)

With the patient lying supine, the manipulator applies point-pressing with the tip of the thumb or middle finger to Qihai (CV 6), 1.5 *cun* below the umbilicus, and Guanyuan (CV 4), 3 *cun* below the umbilicus, each for thirty seconds (fig. 2). It is desirable to induce a feeling of soreness and distension radiating to the perineum.

(3) Point-pressing of Sanyinjiao (SP 6) and Yinlingquan (SP 9)

With the patient lying supine, the manipulator, standing to the side, applies point-pressing with the thumb tips to Sanyinjiao (SP 6), 3 *cun* superior to the medial malleolus

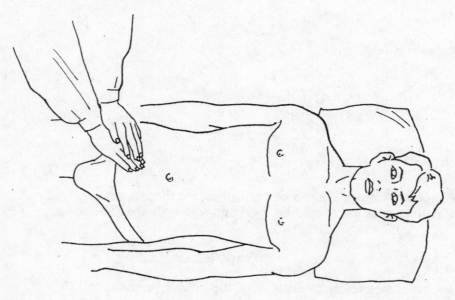

**Fig. 1**

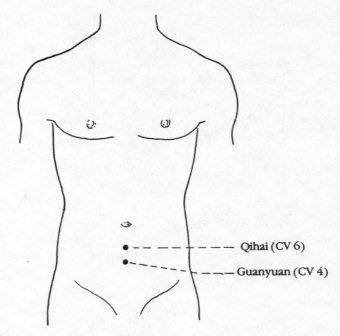

Fig. 2

and just posterior to the tibia, and Yinlingquan (SP 9) in the depression on the medial aspect of the knee, inferior to the medial condyle of the tibia, each for one minute (fig. 3).

(4) Pinching along the spine

With the patient lying prone with the back naked from the coccyx to the seventh cervical vertebra, the manipulator, half clenching the fists with the thumbs stretched upward and the index and middle fingers propped on the patient's coccyx, alternately pushes the right and left hand forward along the spine up to the seventh cervical vertebra while pinching (fig. 4). The manipulation should be repeated 3-5 times, and following three

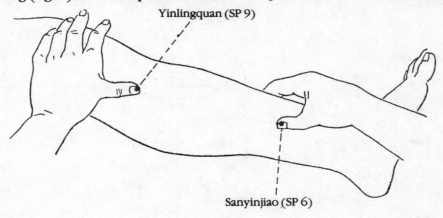

Fig. 3

113

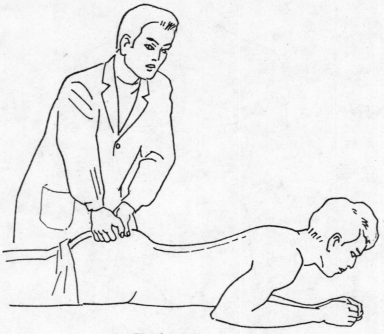

**Fig. 4**

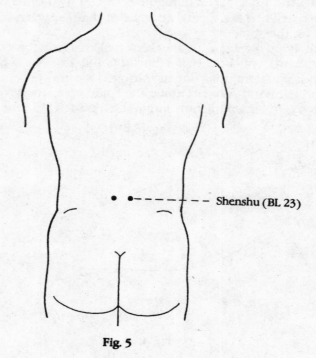

---- Shenshu (BL 23)

**Fig. 5**

114

pushes and pinches, the skin is gently lifted up once. It is desirable to induce slight redness of the skin along the spine.

(5) Pressing-kneading of Shenshu (BL 23)

With the patient taking a sitting position, the manipulator, sitting behind, applies pressing-kneading with thumbs to both Shenshu (CV 23), 1.5 *cun* lateral to the midpoint between the spinous processes of the second and third lumbar vertebrae for one minute (fig. 5).

2. *Self-massage*

(1) Pushing-kneading of the lower abdomen

Lie supine, push and at the same time knead the lateral aspects of the lower abdomen with both palms simultaneously for two minutes (fig. 6).

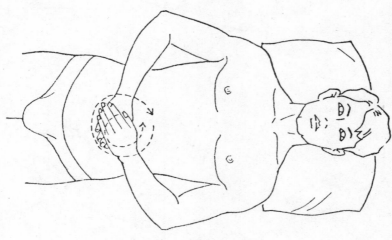

Fig. 6

(2) Stroking of the umbilicus

Lie supine. Placing the centre of the right palm on the umbilicus and overlapping the left palm on the dorsum of the right hand, stroke the umbilicus with both palms simultaneously in circular movements for two minutes (fig. 7).

(3) Rubbing of the lumbo-sacral region

Take a sitting position with the upper trunk slightly bent forward. Place the palms with the fingers closed together on the lumbo-sacral region, and rub the skin up and down for two minutes (fig. 8).

(4) Pressing-kneading of the loins

Take a sitting position. Clenching the fists, apply pressing-kneading with the back part of metacarpophalangeal articulation to the loin of the same side for three minutes (fig. 9).

NB:

(1) Perform the acupoint massage 1-2 times daily.

(2) Be moderate in sexual intercourse and properly alternate work with rest and recreation.

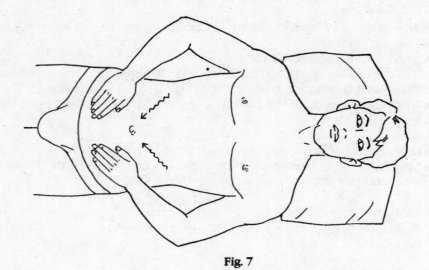

**Fig. 7**

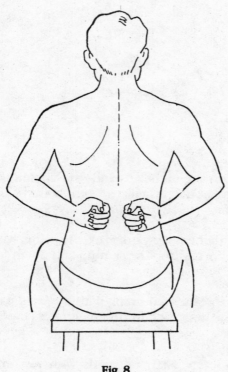

**Fig. 8**

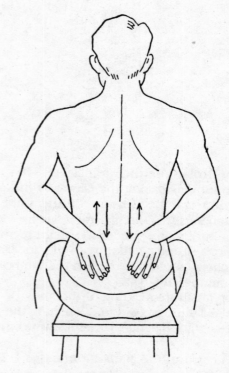

**Fig. 9**

116

# Seminal Emission

Cause: Seminal emission is usually due to overindulgence in sex that leads to the imbalance between the heart and the kidney, or over-drinking that injures the spleen and stomach with consequent downward flow of damp-heat. It may be also due to distension of the urinary bladder or rectum, pressure on the lower abdomen or psychic factors. In most cases, it is a functional disorder.

Main Symptoms: Occasional seminal emission once a week without discomfort or other symptoms is a physiological phenomenon in a male adult unmarried or living apart from his spouse. However, frequent seminal emission is a morbid condition; it is often accompanied by dizziness, listlessness, lassitude, emaciation, loss of memory, aching of the loins, weakness of the legs and impairment of sleep.

Acupoint Massage: This massage has the effect of tonifying the kidney and controlling seminal emission.

[Manipulation]

1. Massage performed by a family member

(1) Point-pressing Guanyuan (CV 4), Zhongji (CV 3), Sanjinjiao (SP 6) and Zusanli (ST 36)

With the patient lying supine, the manipulator, standing to the side, applies point-pressing with the tips of thumbs or middle fingers to Guanyuan (CV 4), 3 cun below the umbilicus, Zhongji (CV 3), 4 cun below the umbilicus, Sanyinjiao (SP 6), 3 cun superior to the tip of the medial malleolus and just posterior to the tibia, and Zusanli (ST 36), 3 cun inferior to the lateral aspect of the knee and one finger's breadth lateral to the tibial crest, each for two minutes (fig. 1).

(2) Grasping-lifting of the lower abdomen

With the patient lying supine, the manipulator, standing to the side, grasps and lifts the abdominal muscles with the hands and then relaxes, working from the upper part to the lower part of the lower abdomen (fig. 2). The manipulation is repeated for two minutes.

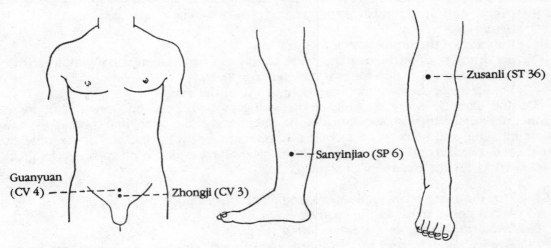

**Fig. 1**

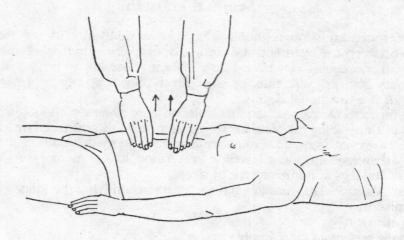

**Fig. 2**

(3) Kneading-pinching of the phalangeal joints of the foot

With the patient lying supine, the manipulator, standing to the side, holds the back of the patient's foot with one hand, and applies kneading and pinching with the thumb, index and middle fingers of the other hand to the phalangeal joints of the foot from the metatarsophalangeal joints to the tip of toes for five minutes.

(4) Pressing-kneading of Xinshu (BL 15), Shenshu (BL 23) and Zhishi (BL 52)

With the patient lying prone, the manipulator, standing to the side, applies pressing-kneading with the thumb tips to Xinshu (BL 15), 1.5 *cun* lateral to the midpoint between the spinous processes of the fifth and sixth thoracic vertebrae, Shenshu (BL 23), 1.5 *cun* lateral to the midpoint between the spinous processes of the second and third lumbar vertebrae, and Zhishi (BL 52), 3 *cun* lateral to the midpoint between the spinous processes of the second and third lumbar vertebrae, each for two minutes (fig. 3).

*2. Self-massage*

(1) Rubbing of the lumbo-sacral region

Take a sitting position. Placing the palms closely against the skin, rub it with force from the loins to the sacral region for two minutes (fig. 4).

(2) Lifting up of the perineum and contracting of the anus

Do the exercise every evening before going to bed. Standing upright, lift up the perineum by pressing with the buttocks and thighs and at the same time contract the anus while inhaling, and relax while exhaling. Repeat this for two minutes. This exercise can build up the health and regulate the physiological function of the nervous system, giving a good effect for the treatment of seminal emission.

NB:

(1) Free the mind of encumbrances, and abstain from masturbation.

(2) Avoid heavy meals in the evening.

(3) Lying on the side is preferred during sleep.

(4) Physical exercise and proper alternation of work with rest and recreation are also of significance.

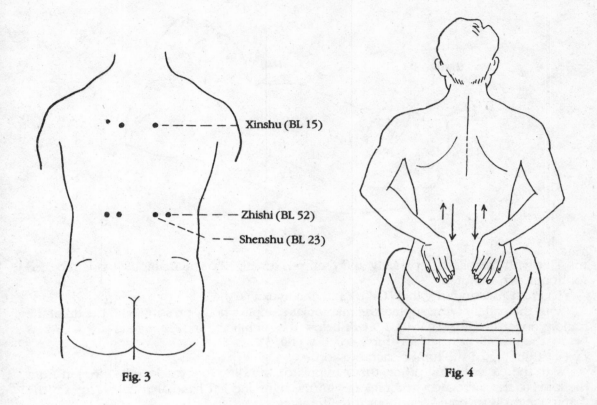

Xinshu (BL 15)

Zhishi (BL 52)

Shenshu (BL 23)

Fig. 3                                                    Fig. 4

# Premature Ejaculation

Cause: Premature ejaculation often happens in conjunction with nervous tension, anxiety, fright, overfatigue, neurasthenia, overindulgence in sex, general debility and convalescence.

Traditional Chinese medicine holds that premature ejaculation is chiefly due to deficiency of the kidney *yin* with exuberant fire.

Main Symptoms: Ejaculation at the very beginning of the sexual intercourse when the penis has just inserted into the vagina or even before the insertion.

Acupoint Massage: This massage has the effect of reinforcing the kidney and quenching the fire.

## [Manipulation]

*1. Massage performed by a family member*

(1) Kneading of the lower abdomen

With the patient lying supine, the manipulator, standing to the side, gently and softly kneads the lower abdomen with the right and left hand alternately from the umbilicus to the pubic symphysis and from the right to the left (fig. 1). The manipulation is repeated for about five minutes.

(2) Grasping-lifting of the abdominal muscles

With the patient lying supine, the manipulator grasps and lifts up the abdominal

119

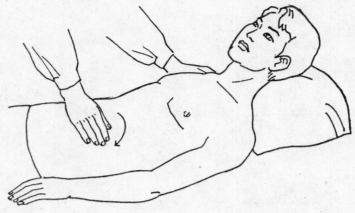

Fig. 1

muscles with the hands separately and then relaxes (fig. 2). The manipulation is repeated for about two minutes.

(3) Point-pressing of Qihai (CV 6) and Guanyuan (CV 4)

With the patient lying supine, the manipulator applies point-pressing with the tip of the middle finger to Qihai (CV 6), 1.5 *cun* below the umbilicus, and Guanyuan (CV 4), 3 *cun* below the umbilicus, each for thirty seconds (fig. 3).

(4) Rubbing of the lumbo-sacral region

With the patient lying prone, the manipulator, standing to the side, rubs the skin from the loins to the sacrococcygeal region with the right and left hand alternately (fig. 4). The manipulation is repeated for about three minutes.

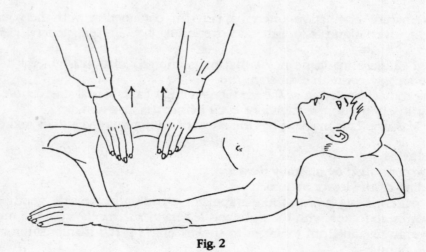

Fig. 2

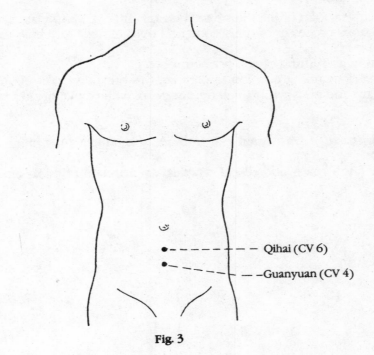

Fig. 3

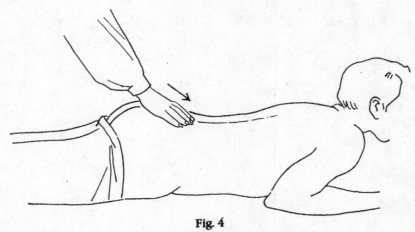

Fig. 4

*2. Self-massage*

(1) Point-pressing of Sanyinjiao (SP 6)

Take a sitting position. Placing the right foot on the left knee, apply point-pressing with the right thumb tip to right Sanyinjiao (SP 6), 3 *cun* superior to the tip of the medial malleolus and just posterior to the tibia (fig. 5). Then apply point-pressing to left Sanyinjiao in the similar way.

(2) Pressing-kneading of Shenshu (BL 23)

Take a sitting position. Clenching fists, apply pressing-kneading with the prominence of the interphalangeal joint of the thumb to Shenshu (BL 23), 1.5 *cun* lateral to the midpoint between the spinous processes of the second and third lumbar vertebrae, each side for two minutes (fig. 6).

(3) Contracting and lifting of the perineum

Take a sitting or standing position to perform this breathing exercise. Contract and lift the scrotum, penis and anus while inhaling, and relax while exhaling. Repeat this for about three minutes.

NB:

(1) Acupoint massage performed 1-2 times daily is effective for premature ejaculation of psychic origin.

(2) Be moderate in sex, and dispel worries. Appropriate physical exercise is recommended.

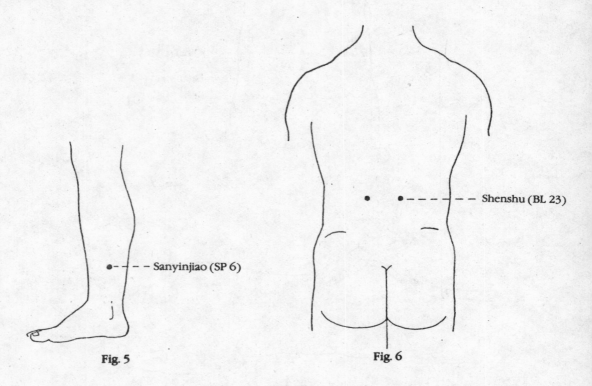

Fig. 5    Fig. 6

# II. Gynecological Diseases

## Chronic Pelvic Inflammation

Cause: Pelvic inflammation is usually due to infections, occurring as a result of delivery, abortion, intercourse during menstruation, after gynecological operation or in patients with lowered resistance. Without due treatment, the chronic stage may follow an acute inflammation. The lesion is often localized to the ovaries, fallopian tubes and pelvic connective tissues.

Main Symptoms: Distension and pain in the lower abdomen, and aching of the lumbo-sacral region, often aggravated after fatigue, sexual intercourse, defecation and around the menstrual period, accompanied by increase of leukorrhea, menostasis or excessive menstrual flow.

Acupoint Massage: This massage has the effect of promoting the blood circulation, removing blood stasis, alleviating inflammation and relieving pain.

[Manipulation]

*1. Massage performed by a family member*

(1) Kneading of the lateral aspects of the lower abdomen

With the patient lying supine, the manipulator, standing to the side, places the palms closely against the lateral aspects of the patient's abdomen, and applies kneading with the right and left palm alternately to the abdomen, beginning gently and softly but with gradual increase in depth (fig. 1). The manipulation is repeated for three minutes.

(2) Point-pressing of Guanyuan (CV 4), Zhongji (CV 3) and Qichong (ST 30)

With the patient lying supine, the manipulator, standing to the side, applies point-pressing with the tip of the middle finger perpendicularly to Guanyuan (CV 4), 3 *cun* below the umbilicus, Zhongji (CV 3), 4 *cun* below the umbilicus, and Qichong (ST 30), 5 *cun* below the umbilicus and 2 *cun* lateral to the anterior midline, each for about thirty seconds (fig. 2). I is desirable to induce a feeling of local soreness and distension.

(3) Pushing of the medial aspect of the leg

With the patient lying supine, the legs stretched straight, the manipulator, standing to the side, places the palms on the medial aspect of the thigh and shank, and applies pushing somewhat forcibly with the right and left palm alternately to and fro in linear movements (fig. 3). The manipulation is repeated for about five minutes.

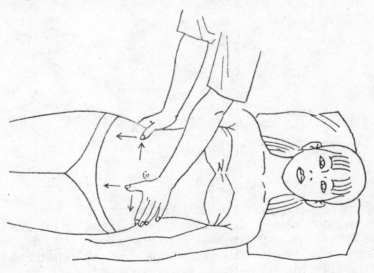

**Fig. 1**

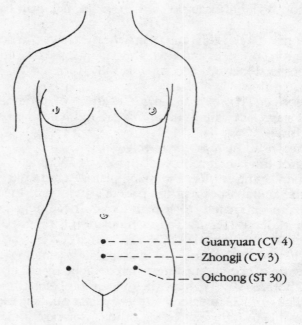

Guanyuan (CV 4)
Zhongji (CV 3)
Qichong (ST 30)

Fig. 2

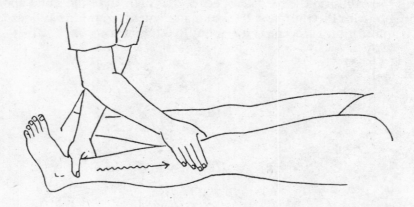

Fig. 3

(4) Point-pressing of Sanyinjiao (SP 6) and Yinlinquan (SP 9)

With the patient lying supine, the manipulator, standing to the side, applies point-pressing with the thumb tips to Sanyinjiao (SP 6), 3 *cun* superior to the tip of the medial malleolus and just posterior to the tibia, and Yinlingquan (SP 9) in the depression of the medial aspect of the knee, inferior to the medial condyle of the tibia, each for about thirty seconds (fig. 4). It is desirable to induce a feeling of numbness and distension radiating downward.

124

## 2. Self-massage

### (1) Stroking of the abdomen

Lie supine with the legs bent. Overlapping the palms and placing them on the middle and lower parts of the abdomen, stroke the abdomen with the palms from the right to the left in clockwise circular movements for about ten minutes (fig. 5). The manipulation should be brisk and soft, with light force at first and then heavier, causing a feeling of warmth of the abdomen.

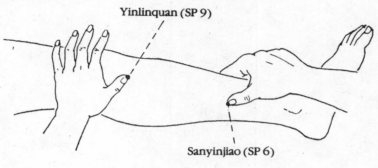

Yinlinquan (SP 9)

Sanyinjiao (SP 6)

Fig. 4

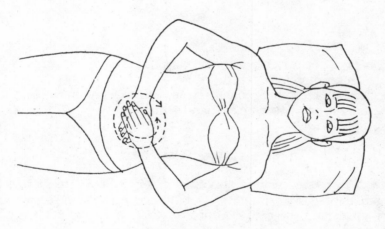

Fig. 5

### (2) Rubbing of the lumbo-sacral region

Take a sitting position with the upper trunk slightly bent forward. Place the palms against the loins with the fingers closed together, and rub the skin forcibly down to the sacral region (fig. 6). Repeat the manipulation for about two minutes to induce slight redness of the skin and a feeling of warmth.

NB:

(1) The massage should be performed twice a day, in the morning and in the evening, but not in the period between the third day before and the fifth day after menstruation.

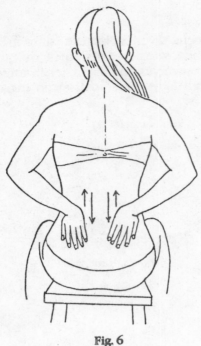

Fig. 6

(2) Application of a hot water bag to the lower abdomen and immersion of the feet into hot water are recommended.

(3) It is important to keep the genitalia clean, be moderate in sexual intercourse, and make proper alternation of work with rest and recreation.

## Menstrual Disorders

Cause: Menstrual disorders include abnormal changes of the menstrual cycle and the amount of menstrual flow. Menstruation is controlled by the hormone secretion of the anterior pituitary gland and the ovary. Abnormal changes in their function will result in menstrual disorders.

According to traditional Chinese medicine, the basic mechanisms of menstrual disorders are heat in the blood that causes bleeding, and deficiency of *qi* with failure of the Thoroughfare and Conception vessels to control menstruation. The common causes are anxiety, overfatigue, colds, indulgence in sex, poor menstrual hygiene and other diseases.

Main Symptoms: Irregular menstrual cycles, either late or early, abnormal amount of menstrual flow, either scanty or profuse, sometimes with continuous dripping, and abnormal colour and viscosity of the menstrual blood, accompanied by distension of the lower abdomen, aching of the loins, irritability, dizziness, cardiac palpitation and insomnia.

Acupoint Massage: This massage has the effect of reinforcing the *qi*, nourishing the blood and expelling pathogenic cold from the meridians.

## [Manipulation]

*1. Massage performed by a family member*

(1) Pushing and shoving of the back along the Bladder Meridian

With the patient lying prone, the manipulator, standing to the side, pushes and shoves the back with the right and left palm alternately from the waist upward along the path of Bladder Meridian (fig. 1). The manipulation is repeated for about five minutes.

(2) Kneading-rubbing of Shangliao (BL 31), Ciliao (BL 32), Zhongliao (BL 33) and Xialiao (BL 34)

With the patient lying prone, the manipulator, standing to the side, supports the patient's waist with one hand and places the other palm closely against the skin at Shangliao (BL 31), Ciliao (BL 32), Zhongliao (BL 33) and Xialiao (BL 34), kneading and

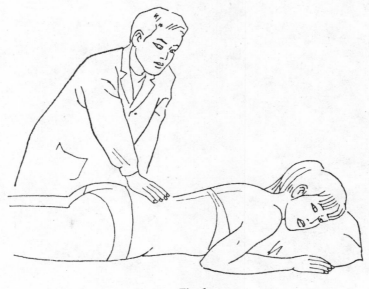

Fig. 1

rubbing the skin down to the area lateral to the coccyx (fig. 2). The manipulation is repeated for about three minutes.

(3) Point-pressing of Guanyuan (CV 4)

With the patient lying supine, the manipulator, standing to the side, applies point-pressing with the middle finger perpendicularly to Guanyuan (CV 4), 3 *cun* below the umbilicus for about thirty seconds to induce a feeling of local aching and distension (fig. 3).

(4) Point-pressing of Xuehai (SP 10)

With the patient lying supine, the manipulator, standing to the side, applies point-pressing with the tip of a thumb perpendicularly to Xuehai (SP 10), 2 *cun* superior to the medial border of the patella, each side for about thirty seconds (fig. 4). It is desirable to induce a feeling of local aching and distension.

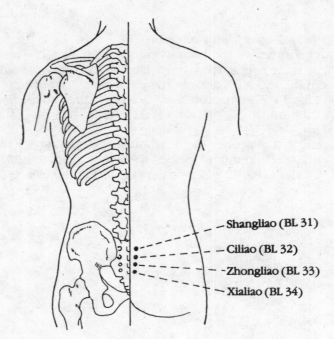

Shangliao (BL 31)

Ciliao (BL 32)

Zhongliao (BL 33)

Xialiao (BL 34)

Fig. 2

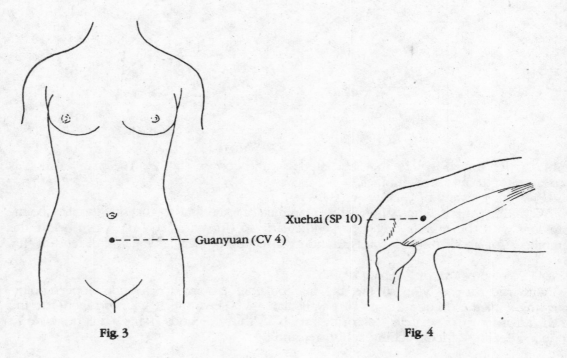

Guanyuan (CV 4)

Xuehai (SP 10)

Fig. 3                                    Fig. 4

(5) Point-pressing of Sanyinjiao (SP 6)

With the patient lying supine, the manipulator, standing to the side, applies point-pressing with the tip of a middle finger perpendicularly to Sanyinjiao (SP 6), 3 *cun* superior to the tip of the medial malleolus and just posterior to the tibia, for about thirty seconds (fig. 5). It is desirable to induce a feeling of local distension and numbness.

*2. Self-massage*

(1) Kneading-rubbing of the abdomen

Lie supine with the legs bent. Overlapping the palms and placing them on the abdomen, knead and rub the lower and middle parts of the abdomen around the umbilicus from the right to the left in clockwise circular movements (fig. 6). The manipulation should be brisk and soft with light force at first and then heavier, inducing a feeling of local warmth.

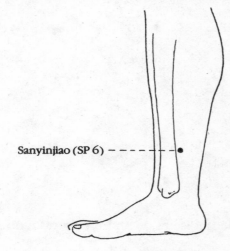

Sanyinjiao (SP 6)

Fig. 5

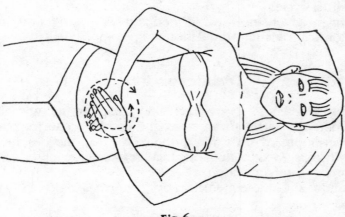

Fig. 6

(2) Point-pressing of Neiguan (PC 6)

Take any position. Apply point-pressing with the right and left thumbs to left and right Neiguan (PC 6) respectively for about thirty seconds. Neiguan (PC 6) is located on the anterior aspect of the forearm, 2 *cun* superior to the midpoint of the wrist crease (fig. 7).

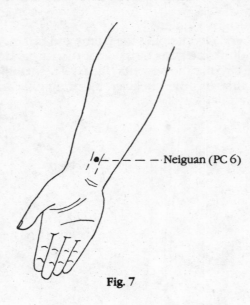

Neiguan (PC 6)

**Fig. 7**

It is desirable to induce a feeling of local distension and numbness radiating to the elbow and upper arm.

NB:

(1) It is best to start the acupoint massage on the tenth day after menstruation, performing it once daily and continuing it until the menstrual onset. Repeat the massage after the next menstrual cycle.

(2) Menstrual hygiene, avoidance of cold food and stimulating food, such as chilli and liquor, and prevention from mental stimulation are recommended.

## Dysmenorrhea

Cause: Dysmenorrhea refers to severe pain taking place around and during menstruation. Primary dysmenorrhea, starting from menarche, usually occurs in young women with nervousness or maldevelopment or flexion of the uterus that impedes the menstrual flow. Secondary dysmenorrhea is a symptom of organic diseases of the reproductive organs, such as endometriosis, tumor or inflammation.

According to traditional Chinese medicine, dysmenorrhea is due to impairment of the flow of *qi* and blood.

Main Symptoms: Dysmenorrhea usually occurs one or two days before the menstruation or on the first day of menstrual onset, and becomes less severe and vanishes during the

130

menstruation. The pain is localized in the lower abdomen, sometimes radiating to the loins and perineum. In severe cases, dysmenorrhea is accompanied by nausea, vomiting, headaches, dizziness and even pallor and cold sweats.

Acupoint Massage: This massage has the effect of promoting the flow of *qi* and blood, regulating menstruation and relieving pain.

**[Manipulation]**

*1. Massage performed by a family member*

(1) Grasping-lifting of the lower abdomen

With the patient lying supine with the hips and legs bent, the manipulator, standing to the side, grasps and at the same time lifts the abdominal skin with the thumb and four fingers of both hands, gradually moving the hands down to the pubic symphysis (fig. 1). The manipulation is repeated 5-7 times.

(2) Pressing of the shank

With the patient lying supine, and manipulator, standing to the right side, applies pressing to the medial aspect of the left shank with the tips of both thumbs, moving from the knee down to the ankle (fig. 2). The manipulation is repeated for about two minutes.

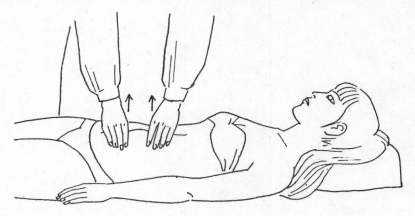

Fig. 1

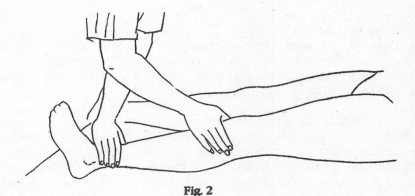

Fig. 2

It is desirable to induce a feeling of local aching and distension radiating to the foot. Similar manipulation is then performed on the right shank.

(3) Pressing-kneading of the back

With the patient lying prone, the manipulator applies pressing-kneading with the right and left palm alternately to the patient's back from the upper part to the lumbo-sacral region along the sides of the spine (fig. 3). The manipulation is repeated for five minutes.

(4) Point-pressing of Sanyinjiao (SP 6)

With the patient lying supine, the manipulator, standing to the side, applies point-pressing with the tip of the middle finger to Sanyinjiao (SP 6), 3 *cun* superior to the tip of the medial malleolus and just posterior to the tibia, for about thirty seconds (fig. 4). It is desirable to induce a feeling of local distension and numbness.

57

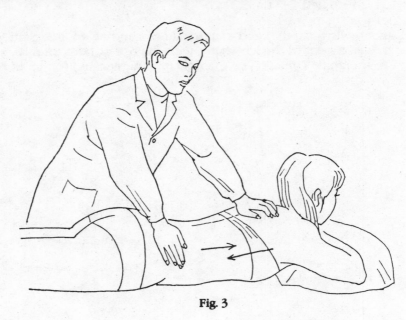

Fig. 3

(5) Point-pressing of Xuehai (SP 10)

With the patient lying supine, the manipulator, standing to the side, applies point-pressing with the thumb perpendicularly to Xuehai (SP 10), 2 *cun* superior to the medial border of the patella, each side for thirty seconds (fig. 5). It is desirable to induce a feeling of local aching and distension.

*2. Self-massage*

(1) Kneading-stroking of the abdomen

Lie supine with the hips and legs bent. Overlapping the palms and placing them on the abdomen, knead and stroke the middle and lower parts of the abdomen around the umbilicus from the right to the left in clockwise circular movements (fig. 6). Repeat the kneading-stroking for ten minutes; the manipulation should be brisk and soft with the force light at first and then heavier.

132

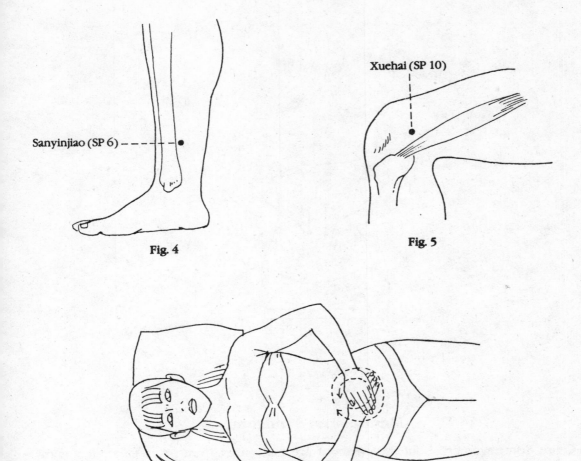

Sanyinjiao (SP 6)

Fig. 4

Xuehai (SP 10)

Fig. 5

Fig. 6

(2) Rubbing of the lumbo-sacral region

Take a sitting position with the fingers closed together and stretched straight. Placing the palms closely against the skin of the lumbo-sacral region, rub from the loins down to the sacro-coccygeal region (fig. 7). Repeat the rubbing for about three minutes.

NB:

(1) Diagnosis should be made by gynecological examination before acupoint massage.

(2) It is appropriate to start the massage once daily on the seventh day after the menstruation, continuing it until three days before the next menstrual onset for 2-3 menstrual cycles.

(3) Keep good menstrual hygiene, protect the warmth of the abdomen, and avoid mental stimulation and overfatigue.

133

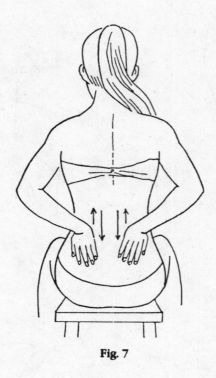

Fig. 7

## Menopausal Syndrome

Cause: Some women about fifty years of age may suffer from neuro-endocrinological disorders, particularly disorders of the antonomic nervous system around climacterium owing to the reduction of ovarian function.

According to traditional Chinese medicine, in women about fifty years of age the Conception and Thoroughfare vessels become devoid of blood and the kidney *qi* is in a state of deficiency with an imbalance of *yin* and *yang*, and hence the menopause takes place.

Main Symptoms: Amenorrhea or irregular menstruation with excessive menstrual flow or continuous dripping of blood, accompanied by dizziness, tinnitus, palpitation, insomnia, irritability, forgetfulness, excessive sweating, lassitude, lumbago, abdominal distension or even abnormal emotional changes.

Acupoint Massage: This massage has the effect of nourishing the kidney *yin* and regulating the Conception and Thoroughfare vessels.

[Manipulation]

*1. Massage performed by a family member*

(1) Pinching along the spine

With the patient lying prone with the back naked from the nape to the coccyx, the manipulator, standing to the side and half clenching the fists naturally with the thumbs

134

stretched out and the index and middle fingers propped on the patient's coccyx, pushes the right and left hand forward alternately while pinching until reaching the seventh cervical vertebra (fig. 1). During manipulation, after three pushes and pinches, there is an uplifting of the skin. It is desirable to induce mild redness of the skin along the spine.

(2) Rubbing of the lumbo-sacral region

With the patient lying prone, the manipulator, standing to the side, supports the patient's waist with one hand and places the other hand closely against the patient's lumbo-sacral region, rubbing the skin with pressure upward and downward or rightward and leftward in linear movements briskly and rapidly to induce local warmth (fig. 2).

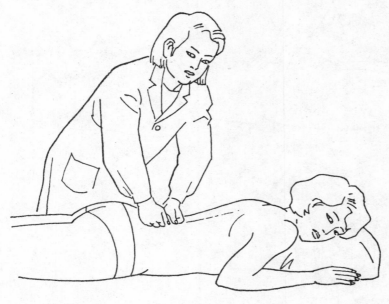

Fig. 1

(3) Point-pressing of Zusanli (ST 36)

With the patient lying supine, the manipulator applies point-pressing with the thumbs to Zusanli (ST 36), 3 *cun* inferior to the lateral aspect of the knee and one finger's breadth lateral to the tibial crest, for about thirty seconds (fig. 3).

(4) Point-pressing of Sanyinjiao (SP 6)

With the patient lying supine, the manipulator applies point-pressing with the thumbs to Sanyinjiao (SP 6), 3 *cun* superior to the tip of the medial malleolus, for thirty seconds (fig. 4).

2. *Self-massage*

(1) Stroking of the face

Rub the palms warm. Stroke the face by the sides of the nose, around the orbits, along the cheeks and near the ears (Fig. 5). Repeat the stroking for about two minutes.

135

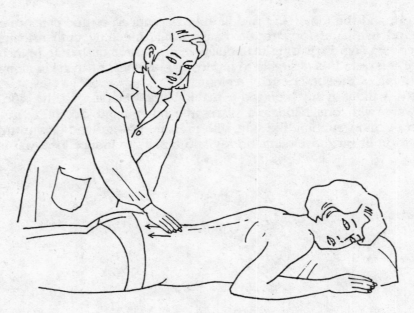

**Fig. 2**

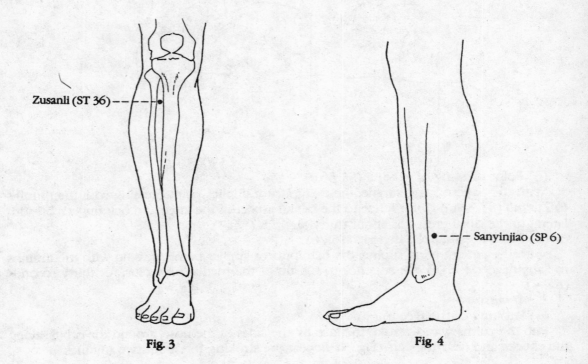

Zusanli (ST 36) ----------•

**Fig. 3**

•---- Sanyinjiao (SP 6)

**Fig. 4**

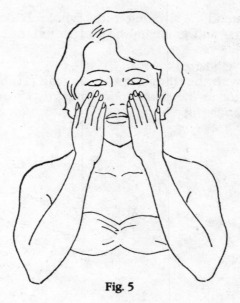

Fig. 5

(2) Stroking of the head

Slightly bend the fingers and keep them separate. Inserting the fingers into the hair on the scalp, stroke the scalp to and fro gently as if dressing or washing the hair, continuing this for about two minutes (fig. 6).

(3) Squeezing-lifting of the nape

Crossing the fingers and holding the nape with the hands, slightly bend the head backward and then squeeze and lift the nape for about one minute (fig. 7).

(4) Stroking of the abdomen

Lie supine with the legs bent. Overlapping the palms, stroke the middle and lower parts of the abdomen with the palms around the umbilicus in clockwise movements for about

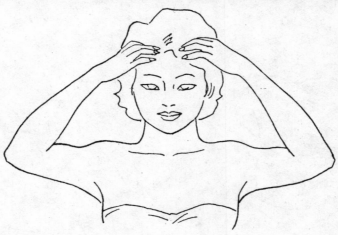

Fig. 6

five minutes, and then extend the stroking to the whole abdomen for about two minutes with the force light at first and gradually heavier to induce a feeling of warmth in the abdomen (fig. 8).

(5) Point-pressing of Neiguan (PC 6)

Apply point-pressing with the thumb tips to Neiguan (PC 6) on the anterior aspect of the forearm, 2 *cun* superior to the midpoint of the wrist crease between the radius and ulna, for about thirty seconds (fig. 9).

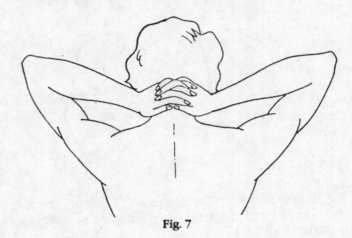

Fig. 7

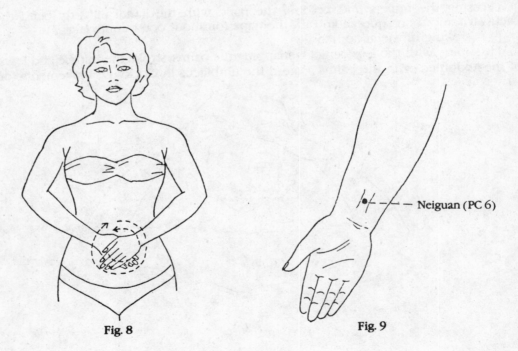

Fig. 8

Neiguan (PC 6)

Fig. 9

NB:

(1) Perform acupoint massage 1-2 times daily for 12 days and then once every other day until the symptoms disappear. Generally, the symptoms will be lessened after 3-5 massages and relieved after 30 massages.

(2) Appropriate physical exercise, alternation of work with rest and recreation and avoidance of mental stimulation are recommended.

## Amenorrhea

Cause: Amenorrhea is defined as no onset of menstruation in a girl over 18 years of age or interruption of menstruation for more than three months in a woman not in pregnancy, lactation or menopause due to age. It has multiple causes related to endocrine, nervous and psychic factors.

According to traditional Chinese medicine, amenorrhea due to exhaustion of blood is caused by multiparity, overcontemplation, weak constitution or debility after a disease, and amenorrhea due to stagnation of blood is caused by exposure to cold and depression.

Main Symptoms: No menstruation after the due time, accompanied by aching of the back, general weakness, indigestion, depression, dizziness, insomnia, a feeling of suffocation in the chest and fidgetiness.

Acupoint Massage: This massage has the effect of promoting the flow of *qi* and blood.

**[Manipulation]**

*1. Massage performed by a family member*

(1) Pushing of the back

With the patient lying prone, the manipulator, standing to the side, applies pushing with the right and left hand alternately to the back along the Bladder Meridian from the upper part down to the lumbo-sacral region (fig. 1). Repeat it for about three minutes.

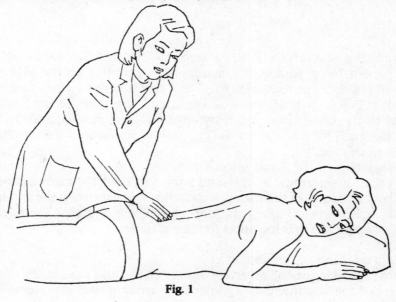

Fig. 1

(2) Pressing-kneading of Ganshu (BL 18), Pishu (BL 20) and Shenshu(BL 23)

With the patient lying prone, the manipulator, standing to the side, applies pressing-kneading with the thumb tips to Ganshu (BL 18), 1.5 *cun* lateral to the midpoint between the spinous processes of ninth and tenth thoracic vertebrae, Pishu (BL 20), 1.5 *cun* lateral to the midpoint between the spinous processes of the eleventh and twelfth thoracic vertebrae, and Shenshu (BL 23), 1.5 *cun* lateral to the midpoint between the second and third lumbar vertebrae, each for about thirty seconds (fig. 2). It is desirable to induce a feeling of local aching and distension.

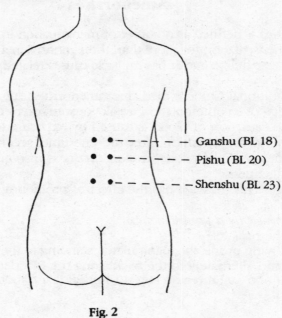

**Fig. 2**

(3) Point-pressing of Xuehai (SP 10), Zusanli (ST 36) and Sanyinjiao (SP 6)

With the patient lying supine, the manipulator, standing to the side, applies point-pressing with the thumb tips to Xuehai (SP 10), 2 *cun* superior to the medial border of the patella, Zusanli (ST 36), 3 *cun* inferior to the lateral aspec of the knee and one finger's breadth lateral to the tibial crest, and Sanyinjiao (SP 6), 3 *cun* superior to the tip of the medial malleolus, each for thirty seconds (fig. 3). It is desirable to induce a feeling of local distension and numbness.

(4) Grasping-lifting of the Conception Vessel

With the patient lying supine with the hips and legs bent, the manipulator, placing both hands on the lateral aspects of the patient's abdomen and squeezing the abdominal muscles by pushing the hands inward along the Conception Vessel, grasps the muscles and then relaxes (fig. 4). Repeat the manipulation for one minute.

*2. Self-massage*

(1) Kneading-stroking of the abdomen

Lie supine with the legs bent. Overlapping the palms and placing them on the middle and lower parts of the abdomen, apply kneading-stroking with the palms from the right

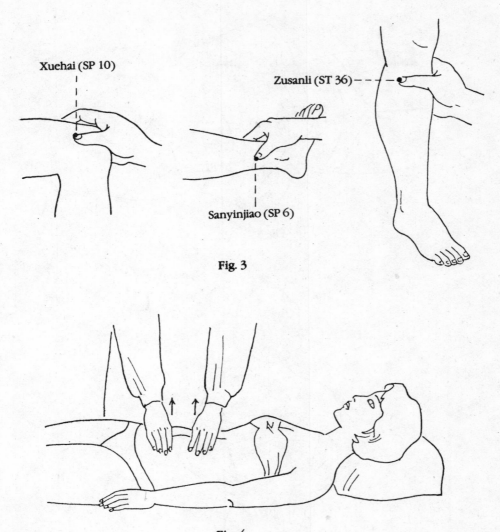

Xuehai (SP 10)

Zusanli (ST 36)

Sanyinjiao (SP 6)

Fig. 3

Fig. 4

to the left in clockwise circular movements repeatedly for about ten minutes (fig. 5). The manipulation should be soft with light force at first and then heavier until there is a feeling of warmth in the abdomen.

(2) Rubbing of the lumbo-sacral region

Take a sitting position with the upper trunk slightly bent forward. Placing the palms against the loins with the fingers closed together, rub the skin with force down to the sacral region (fig. 6). Repeat the manipulation for about two minutes to induce a feeling of local warmth.

(3) Point-pressing of Hegu (LI 4)

Take a sitting or lying position. Apply point-pressing with the right and left thumb tip alternately to the opposite Hegu (LI 4) between the first and second metacarpal bones and

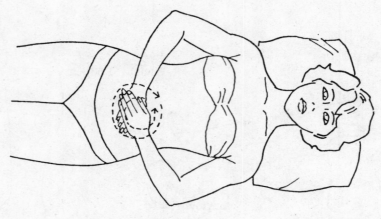

Fig. 5

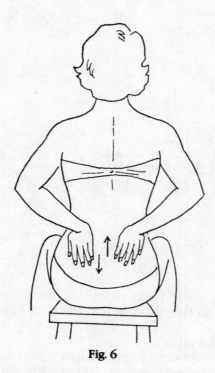

Fig. 6

on the radial aspect of the second metacarpal, each for about one minute (fig. 7). It is desirable to induce a feeling of local distension and heaviness radiating to the fingers.

NB:

(1) Acupoint massage performed twice a day in the morning and in the evening is effective for amenorrhea caused by psychic factors.

142

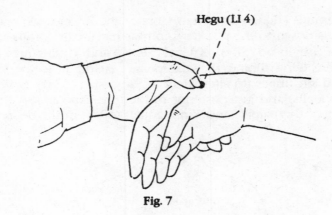

Hegu (LI 4)

Fig. 7

(2) Diagnosis should be made by gynecological examination before acupoint massage begins.

(3) Appropriate physical exercise, avoidance of mental tension and keeping a calm mood are recommended.

## Excessive Leukorrhea

Cause: Excessive whitish discharge from the vagina is often caused by infections such as vaginitis, cervicitis, endometritis and inflammation of the pelvis, but it can also result from weak constitution, constipation and emotional stimuli.

According to traditional Chinese medicine, excessive leukorrhea is due to weakness of the Conception Vessel and failure of the Belt Vessel to control the vaginal discharge, with consequent downward flow of damp-heat.

Main Symptoms: Increased vaginal secretion, abnormal in colour and smell, accompanied by genital pruritus, aching and weakness of the loins or distension and pain in the lower abdomen.

Acupoint Massage: This massage has the effect of regulating the Conception and Belt vessels, removing dampness and arresting the vaginal discharge.

[Manipulation]

*1. Massage performed by a family member*

(1) Pressing-kneading of Daimai (GB 26)

With the patient lying on the side, the manipulator applies pressing-kneading with the ventral aspect of the thumb to Daimai (GB 26), a junction point of the Gallbladder Meridian and the Belt Vessel, located inferior to the anterior end of the eleventh rib and at the same level with the umbilicus, working each side for about one minute (fig. 1), and then pressing-kneading with the fingers of the right and left hand alternately around the waist at the level of Daimai (GB 26) for about five minutes.

(2) Stroking and vibrating of the lower abdomen

With the patient lying supine, the manipulator, standing to the side, strokes the patient's lower abdomen with the right and left palm alternately from the right to the left repeatedly

143

for about two minutes (fig. 2); and then vibrates the lower abdomen along the midline from the umbilicus down to the pubic symphysis repeatedly for about one minute.

(3) Pressing of Sanyinjiao (SP 6), Xuehai (SP 10) and Yinlingquan (SP 9)

With the patient lying supine, the manipulator, standing to the side, applies pressing with the right and left finger tip alternately to Sanyinjiao (SP 6), 3 *cun* superior to the tip of the medial malleolus and just posterior to the tibia, Xuehai (SP 10), 2 *cun* superior to the medial border of the patella, and Yinlingquan (SP 9) in the depression on the medial

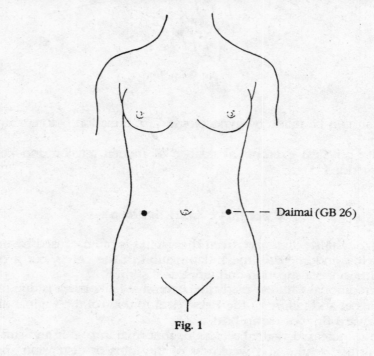

Daimai (GB 26)

**Fig. 1**

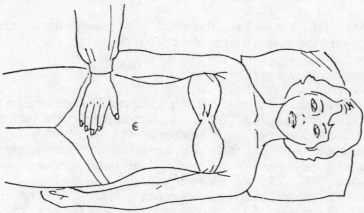

**Fig. 2**

aspect of the knee, inferior to the medial condyle of the tibia, each for one minute (fig. 3).

(4) Pushing-kneading of the lumbo-sacral region

With the patient lying prone, the manipulator, standing to the side, pushes while kneading with the right and left palm alternately from the loins to the sacral region and from the left to the right (fig. 4). Repeat the manipulation for about five minutes.

2. *Self-massage*

(1) Rubbing and striking of the lower abdomen

Lie supine with the hips and legs slightly bent. Placing the palms on the lateral aspects of the lower abdomen, rub and stroke the skin from the upper to the lower and from the lateral to the medial (fig. 5). Repeat the manipulation for about three minutes.

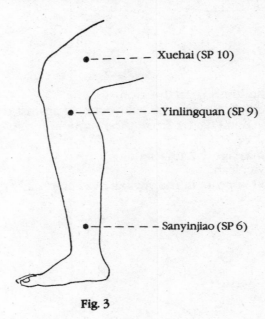

Fig. 3

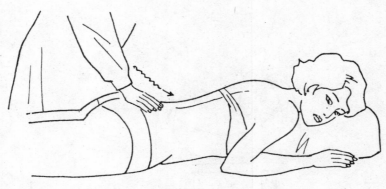

Fig. 4

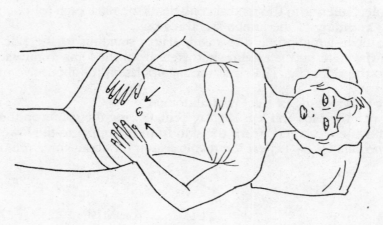

**Fig. 5**

(2) Rubbing of the lumbo-sacral region

Take a sitting position. Placing the palms closely against the skin, rub it from the loins down to the sacral region (fig. 6). Repeat the rubbing for about five five minutes.

NB:

(1) Perform the massage 1-2 times a day.

(2) Keep the vulva clean.

(3) If pus or blood appears in the vaginal discharge, early gynecological examination is necessary.

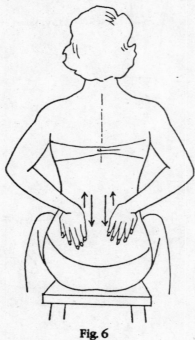

**Fig. 6**

# III. Pediatric Diseases

## Bronchitis in Children

Cause: Bronchitis is a common infectious disease of the upper respiratory tract in children, mostly caused by a mixed viral and bacterial infection. Colds without due treatment may turn to bronchitis. Children with rickets, malnutrition, vitamin deficiency or weak constitution with lowered resistance are apt to contract bronchitis.

Main Symptoms: Running nose, sneezing, fever and coughing at the early stage. The cough is paroxysmal, with or without expectoration of whitish frothy or viscid sputum. If the patient is not treated in due time, chronic bronchitis or even asthmatic bronchitis will develop.

Acupoint Massage: This massage has the effect of dispelling wind, inducing diaphoresis and relieving cough.

**[Manipulation]**

(1) Tonification of the spleen

The child takes a sitting position. The manipulator, holding the child's left thumb with one hand and placing the other hand on the ventral aspect of the thumb, pushes the thumb from the root to the tip for one minute (fig. 1). Then apply the same manipulation to the right thumb.

(2) Massage of the "Inner Eight Diagrams"

The circle of "Inner Eight Diagrams" is located on the palm, with the centre of the palm as the centre of the circle and the distance between the centre and the root of the middle finger as the radius. The child takes a sitting position, and the manipulator holds the child's right palm with one hand, massages the palm with the other hand along the "Inner Eight Diagrams" in circular movements for one minute. Then apply similar manipulation to the left palm (fig. 2).

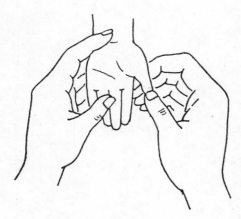

**Fig. 1**

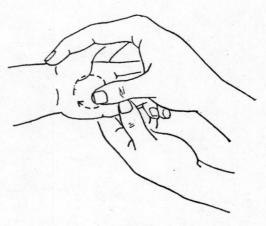

**Fig. 2**

(3) Removing of heat from the Lung Meridian

The child takes a sitting position. The manipulator, holding the child's right palm with one hand and placing the other hand on the ventral aspect of the ring finger, pushes the hand from the tip of the ring finger to its root repeatedly for one minute. Then apply the same manipulation on the left ring finger (fig. 3).

(4) Shoving of Tiantu (CV 22)

Tiantu (CV 22) is located in the centre of the suprasternal fossa. With the child taking a sitting position, the manipulator places the tip of the middle finger on Tiantu (CV 22) and applies kneading in circular motion for one minute (fig. 4).

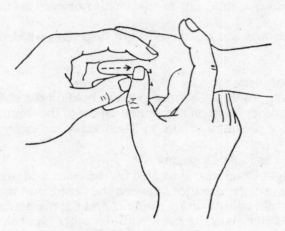

Fig. 3

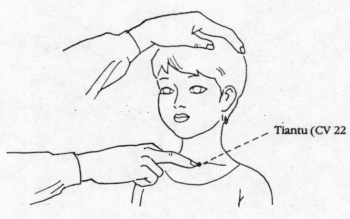

Tiantu (CV 22

Fig. 4

(5) Up-pushing of Tianmen

Tianmen is the line joining the midpoint between the eyebrows and the midpoint of the anterior hairline. With the child taking a sitting position, the manipulator pushes Tianmen straight upward with the ventral aspect of both thumbs for one minute (fig. 5).

(6) Pressing-kneading of Feishu (BL 13))

With the child taking a sitting position, the manipulator, sitting behind, applies pressing-kneading with the thumb tips to Feishu (BL 13), 1.5 *cun* lateral to the midpoint between the spinous processes of the third and fourth thoracic vertebrae, for about one minute (fig. 6).

(7) Pinching alone the spine

Let the child lie prone with the back naked from the seventh cervical vertebra to the coccyx. The manipulator, standing to the side and half clenching the fists with the thumbs stretched out and the index and middle fingers propped on the coccyx, pushes the right and left hand forward alternately up to the seventh cervical vertebra while pinching, and after three pushes and pinches lifts the skin once (fig. 7). It is desirable to induce mild redness of the skin along the spine.

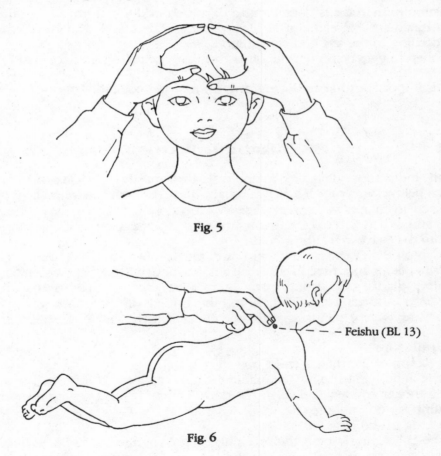

Fig. 5

Fig. 6

— Feishu (BL 13)

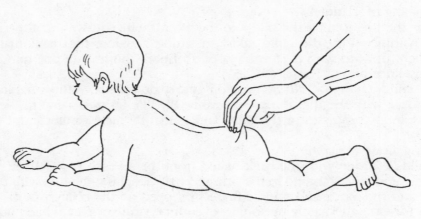

**Fig. 7**

NB:

(1) Acupoint massage is done twice a day, each in the morning and in the evening, a course of treatment consisting of 12 days, or more if necessary. The force of manipulation varies according to the age and constitution.

(2) If there is aggravation of the disease, it is advised to visit a doctor and receive drug therapy.

(3) It is important to keep the child warm to avoid cold, the latter usually aggravating bronchitis.

## Infantile Indigestion

Infantile indigestion, also called infantile diarrhea, mostly occurs in summer and autumn in children below two years of age. It is usually due to imperfect development of the spleen and stomach in infants with weak digestive function. It may also result from improper feeding, eating of raw, cold or unsanitary food, bacterial or viral infection, colds and exposure to excessive warmth or cold.

Main Symptoms: Diarrhea, frequent bowel movements with loose watery stools, greenish yellow in colour and mixed with small amount of whitish or yellowish mucus; in severe cases, watery diarrhea occurring many times a day, accompanied by nausea, vomiting, anorexia, fever, restlessness, listlessness and impairment of consciousness.

Acupoint Massage: This massage has the effect of invigorating the spleen and relieving diarrhea.

[Manipulation]

(1) Kneading of the thenar eminence

With the child lying supine, the manipulator, holding the child's wrist with one hand, kneads the thenar eminence close to the dorso-ventral boundary with the ventral aspect of the thumb for one minute (fig. 1).

(2) Pushing of the large intestine

With the child lying supine, the manipulator, holding the child's index finger with one hand and placing the ventral aspect of the thumb of the other hand on the radial aspect

150

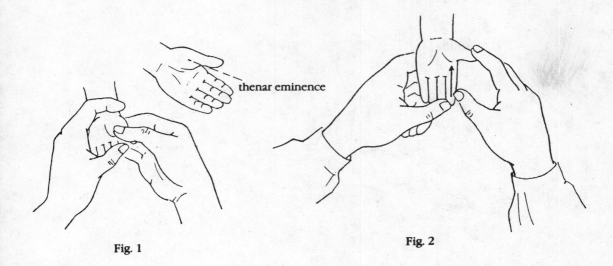

thenar eminence

Fig. 1

Fig. 2

of the patient's index finger, pushes the thumb from the tip of the index finger to its root for one minute (fig. 2).

(3) Stroking of the abdomen

With the child lying supine, the manipulator, sitting to the side, places the ventral aspect of the index, middle, ring and small fingers or the back part of the palm on the child's abdomen, gently, softly and rhythmically stroking the abdomen around the umbilicus for three minutes (fig. 3).

(4) Kneading of the coccyx tip

With the child lying prone, the manipulator, supporting the child's buttocks with one hand, kneads the tip of the child's coccyx with the ventral aspect of the middle finger of the other hand for one minute (fig. 4).

(5) Pinching of the spine

With the child lying prone, the back naked to the inferior border of the coccyx, the manipulator, bending the fingers naturally and propping the index and middle fingers on

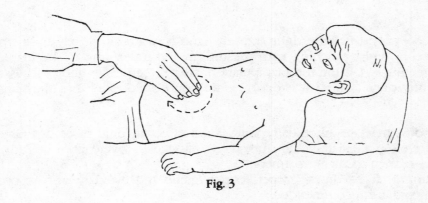

Fig. 3

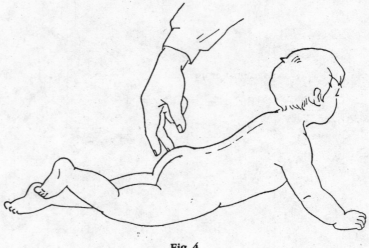

**Fig. 4**

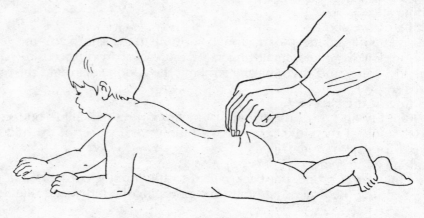

**Fig. 5**

the child's coccyx, pushes the right and left hand forward alternately up to the seventh cervical vertebra while pinching with the thumb and index finger. The manipulation is repeated three times. During the manipulation, after three pushes and pinches, the skin is lifted up gently once (fig. 5). It is desirable to induce mild redness of the skin along the spine.

NB:

(1) Acupoint massage once daily gives good effect in mild cases of indigestion; the symptoms are often alleviated after three days' massage. In severe cases, it is advised to see a doctor and receive medical treatment.

(2) Feeding at fixed times, proper food hygiene and avoidance of exposure of the abdomen to cold are recommended.

# Enuresis in Children

Cause: Enuresis in children refers to involuntary discharge of the urine at night and during sleep in children over three years of age. It has multiple causes. Acupoint massage has good effect for functional enuresis due to impaired control of urination, such as enuresis due to mental tension, overfatigue, too quickly falling to sleep or the parents' insufficient care for the child to foster the habit of passing the urine at fixed times during the night.

According to traditional Chinese medicine, enuresis in children is chiefly due to constitutional weakness with insufficiency of the kidney *qi* and failure of the urinary bladder to restrain the urine.

Main Symptoms: Involuntary discharge of the urine during sleep once or several times a night, sometimes also accompanied by listlessness and emaciation.

Acupoint Massage: This massage has the effect of tonifying the kidney and restoring voluntary urination function.

## [Manipulation]

(1) Kneading of Qihai (CV 6), Guanyuan (CV 4) and Zhongji (CV 3)

With the child lying supine, the manipulator, standing to the side, applies kneading with the tip of a middle finger to Qihai (CV 6), 1.5 *cun* below the umbilicus, Guanyuan (CV 4), 3 *cun* below the umbilicus, and Zhongji (CV 3), 4 *cun* below the umbilicus, each for about one minute (fig. 1).

(2) Point-pressing of Sanyinjiao (SP 6)

With the child lying supine, the manipulator, holding the child's ankle with one hand, applies point-pressing with the thumb tips to Sanyinjiao (SP 6), 3 *cun* superior to the tip of the medial malleolus and just posterior to the tibia, for about one minute (fig. 2).

(3) Pressing-kneading of Feishu (BL 13), Pishu (BL 20), Shenshu (BL 23) and Pang-guangshu (BL 28)

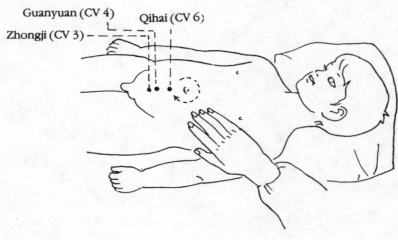

Fig. 1

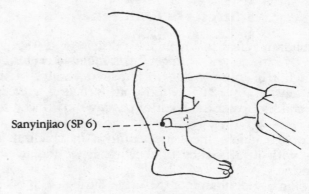

Fig. 2

With the child lying prone, the manipulator, sitting to the side, applies pressing-kneading with both thumb tips simultaneously to bilateral Feishu (CV 13), 1.5 *cun* lateral to the midpoint between the spinous processes of the third and fourth thoracic vertebrae, Pishu (BL 20), 1.5 *cun* lateral to the midpoint between the spinous processes of the eleventh and twelfth thoracic vertebrae, Shenshu (BL 23), 1.5 *cun* lateral to the midpoint between the spinous processes of the second and third lumbar vertebrae, and Pangguangshu (BL 28), 1.5 *cun* lateral to the midpoint between the spinous processes of the second and third sacral vertebrae, each for about one minute (fig. 3).

(4) Pushing of the terminal seven vertebrae

With the child lying prone, the manipulator, holding the child with one hand, pushes the terminal seven vertebrae, i.e., the fourth and fifth lumbar vertebrae together with the sacral vertebrae, from the lower to the upper with the ventral aspect of the thumb for about one minute (fig. 4). It is desirable to induce mild local redness and a feeling of warmth.

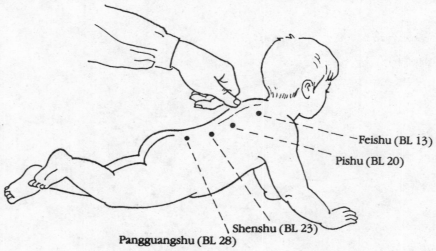

Fig. 3

154

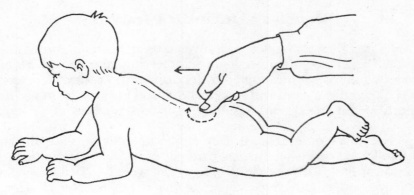

Fig. 4

(5) Tonifying of the kidney

With the child sitting, the manipulator, fixing the child's right small finger with one hand, pushes the ventro-radial aspect of the small finger with the thumb of the other hand from the tip to the root of the small finger (fig. 5). Similar manipulation is then applied to the left small finger.

NB:

(1) Acupoint massage should be performed once every evening before the child goes to bed. During the massage treatment, it is important to train the child to form a habit of passing the urine at fixed times and to awaken the child during the night for urination.

(2) Avoid overfatigue.

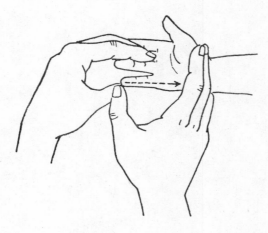

Fig. 5

# Sequelae of Infantile Paralysis

Cause: Infantile paralysis, also called poliomyelitis, is an acute infectious disease caused by the poliovirus. The disease often occurs in summer and autumn. The virus discharged with oral secretions and feces is transmitted by food and direct contact. It enters the human body through the digestive system and nasopharynx, and invades the motor nerve cells of the anterior horn of the spinal cord, resulting in flaccid paralysis of the corresponding muscles.

Main Symptoms: At the onset there usually are fever, and gastro-intestinal and respiratory symptoms, followed by unsymmetrical paralysis of the limbs, more frequently flaccid paralysis of the lower limb with muscle atrophy and lowered surface temperature, as well as deviation of eye and mouth angle, tilting of the head, inability to stand and walk, strephenopodia and equinovarus.

Acupoint Massage: This massage has the effect of promoting blood circulation, removing obstruction from the collaterals and correcting deformities.

[**Manipulation**]

(1) Pressing-kneading of Jianyu (LI 15), Quchi (LI 11), Hegu (LI 4), Fengshi (GB 31), Zusanli (ST 36) and Jiexi (ST 41) of the affected side

With the child lying supine, the manipulator, standing to the side, applies pressing and kneading with the thumb tips to Jianyu (LI 15), in the depression anterior to the end of the shoulder as the arm is in full abduction, Quchi (LI 11), in the depression at the lateral end of the elbow crease as the elbow is flexed, Hegu (LI 4), between the first and second metacarpal bones and on the radial aspect of the second metacarpal, Fengshi (GB 31), on the lateral aspect of the thigh, 7 *cun* superior to the inferior border of the patella, Zusanli (ST 36), 3 *cun* inferior to the lateral aspect of the knee and one finger's breadth lateral to the tibial crest, and Jiexi (ST 41), in the centre of the anterior skin crease of the ankle between the two tendons, each for about one minute (fig. 1).

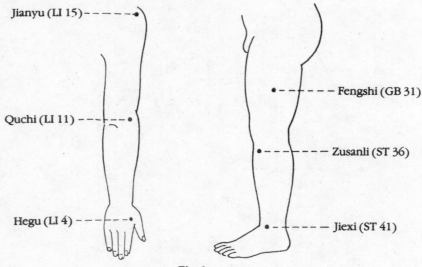

Jianyu (LI 15)

Fengshi (GB 31)

Quchi (LI 11)

Zusanli (ST 36)

Hegu (LI 4)

Jiexi (ST 41)

Fig. 1

156

(2) Pinching-kneading of the affected regions

With the child lying supine, the manipulator, standing to the side, holds the affected limb with one hand, kneading and pinching the affected areas with the other hand from the shoulder to the elbow, wrist and fingertips or from the hip to the knee, ankle and tips of the toes (fig. 2).

(3) Grasping of the affected limb

With the child lying on the side, the manipulator, standing to the side, holds the affected limb with one hand, grasping and pinching the lateral aspect of the limb from the shoulder to the wrist or from the hip to the ankle (fig. 3). The manipulation is repeated for about two minutes.

(4) Point-pressing of Chengfu (BL 36), Weizhong (BL 40) and Kunlun (BL 60)

With the child lying prone, the manipulator, standing to the side, holds the affected limb with one hand and applies point-pressing with the tip of the middle finger of the other hand to Chengfu (BL 36), on the posterior aspect of the thigh, in the centre of the inferior gluteal crease, Weizhong (BL 40), on the posterior aspect of the knee, at the centre of the popliteal skin crease; and Kunlun (BL 60) on the posterior aspect of the lateral malleolus and the anterio-lateral border of the calcaneal tendon, each for one minute (fig. 4).

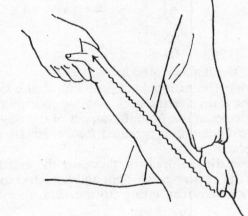

Fig. 2

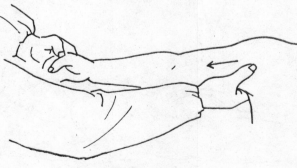

Fig. 3

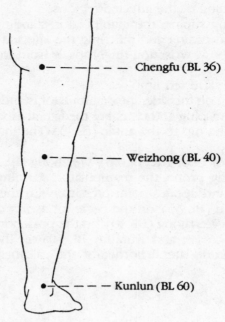

Chengfu (BL 36)

Weizhong (BL 40)

Kunlun (BL 60)

Fig. 4

(5) Pushing-kneading of the Bladder Meridian

With the child lying prone, the manipulator, standing to the side, pushes and at same time kneads the skin with the thumb or the back part of a palm along the Bladder Meridian from the back, loin and buttocks to the posterior aspect of the thigh and the lateral aspect of the shank (fig. 5). The manipulation is repeated for five minutes.

(6) Pinching along the spine

With the child lying prone, the manipulator, propping the index and middle fingers on the child's sacro-coccygeal region, pushes the right and left hand forward alternately while pinching along the Governor Meridian, lifting up the skin once after three pushes and

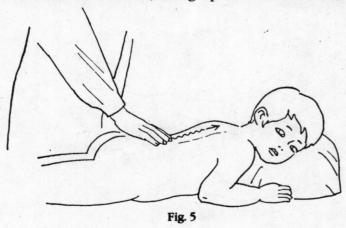

Fig. 5

pinches until the hands reach the seventh cervical vertebra (fig. 6). The manipulation is repeated for 3-5 times.

NB:

(1) Acupoint massage should be done softly and gently with proper force.

(2) In combination with the massage, active and passive motion of the affected limb should be performed under the doctor's guidance to promote the recovery of motor function, increase the muscle strength, prevent muscular atrophy and correct deformity.

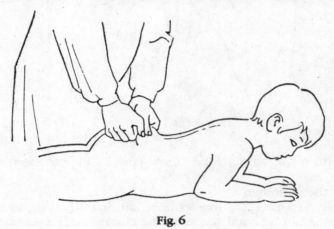

Fig. 6

## Infantile Malnutrition

Cause: Malnutrition often occurs in infants under five years of age whose visceral organs are delicate and digestive functions weak. They are apt to be malnourished if the feeding is improper, the food or milk is unsanitary, too much fatty, sweet or raw and cold food is given, or there is no careful nursing during convalescence, particularly if chronic diarrhea or dysentery is contracted.

Main Symptoms: At the onset there is anorexia, diarrhea with passage of fetid stools and abdominal distension; then occurs emaciation, loss of body weight, distended abdomen with protruded umbilicus, scanty hair, listlessness and even maldevelopment.

Acupoint Massage: This massage has the effect of removing the retained food and invigorating the digestive function.

[Manipulation]

(1) Pushing of the spleen*

With the child lying supine, the manipulator holds the child's wrist with one hand and places the thumb of the other hand on the radial aspect of the child's thumb, pushing from the tip to the root (fig. 1). Repeat the manipulation for two minutes.

(2) Pushing of the "three passes"

With the child lying supine, the manipulator holds the child's forearm with one hand and places the ventral aspect of the thumb of the other hand on the radial aspect of the

---

* The "spleen" in traditional Chinese medicine is believed to be the visceral organ that has the functions of digesting food and absorbing nutrients.

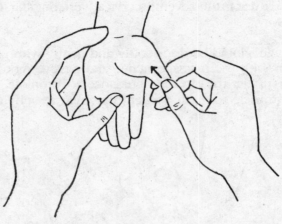

**Fig. 1**

forearm, pushing from the wrist to the elbow (fig. 2). Repeat the manipulation for two minutes.

(3) Stroking of the abdomen

With the child lying supine, the manipulator, sitting to the side, uses the index, middle, ring and small fingers of one hand to stroke the child's abdomen rhythmically, softly and gently around the umbilicus in circular movements clockwise for about two minutes, and then counterclockwise for about two minutes (fig. 3).

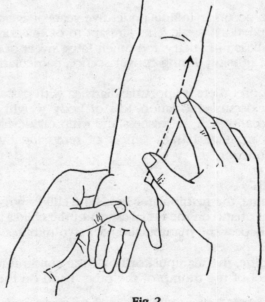

**Fig. 2**

160

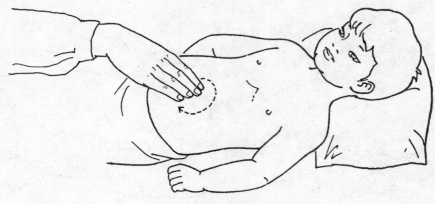

**Fig. 3**

(4) Pressing-kneading of Zusanli (ST 36)

With the child lying supine, the manipulator holds the child's shank with one hand and applies rotary pressing-kneading with the thumb tip to Zusanli (ST 36), 3 *cun* inferior to the lateral aspect of the knee and one finger's breadth lateral to the tibial crest, for about one minute (fig. 4).

(5) Pinching along the spine

With the child lying prone with the back naked to the lower border of the coccyx, the manipulator, bending the fingers naturally and propping the index and middle fingers on the coccyx, pushes the right and left hand forward alternately while pinching with the thumb and index finger up to the seventh thoracic vertebra, and gently lifts up the skin once after three pushes and pinches (fig. 5). It is desirable to induce mild redness of the skin along the spine.

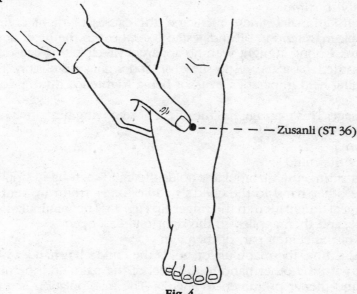

— Zusanli (ST 36)

**Fig. 4**

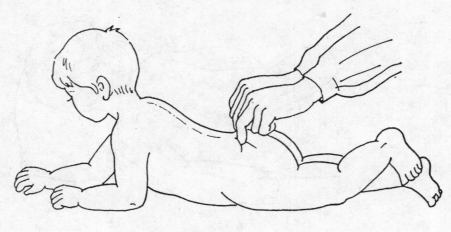

**Fig. 5**

NB:

(1) It is advised to perform acupoint massage once a day and feed the child at fixed times with fixed quantities. Overfeeding, hunger or partiality for a particular kind of food should be avoided.

(2) If malnutrition is due to a chronic disease, the latter should be treated.

## Night Crying of Babies

Cause: A baby with "night crying" is one who has no disease but cries every night on and off or even continuously. This is due to immaturity of the nervous system and a resultant sensitivity to stimuli.

According to traditional Chinese medicine, the causes of night crying in babies are coldness in the spleen, retention of undigested food, heat in the heart and fright.

Main Symptoms: Crying at night with no apparent precipitating cause, accompanied by a flushed face bathed in tears, restlessness or abdominal distension, flexion of limbs, expectation of being held in parent's arms, or being frightened during sleep and crying in a dream.

Acupoint Massage: This massage has the effect of removing heat, invigorating the spleen and inducing tranquilization.

[Manipulation]

(1) Calming of the mind

With the child sitting, the manipulator holds the child's left hand, applies pushing with the thumb of the other hand to the child's middle finger from the ventral aspect of the metacarpophalangeal articulation to the finger tip (fig. 1). The manipulation is repeated for about one minute, and then applied to the right middle finger.

(2) Kneading of the central part of the palm

With the child sitting, the manipulator holds the child's left hand with one hand, and applies kneading with the other hand to the heel of the palm and the midpoint between the hypothenar and thenar prominences (fig. 2). The manipulation is repeated for about two minutes, and then applied to the child's right hand.

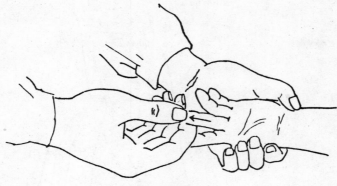

**Fig. 1**

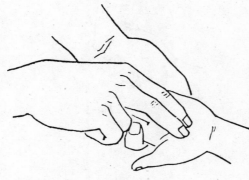

**Fig. 2**

(3) Pushing of the "three passes"

With the child lying supine, the manipulator holds the child's right hand, and applies pushing to the radial aspect of the forearm from the skin crease of the wrist to that of the elbow (fig. 3). The manipulation is repeated for one minute and then applied to the child's left hand.

(4) Stroking of the abdomen

With the child lying supine, the manipulator, sitting to the side, uses the ventral aspect of the index, middle, ring and small fingers or the heel of the palm to stroke the child's abdomen around the umbilicus rhythmically, softly and gently in clockwise circular movements for about two minutes (fig. 4).

(5) Tonifying of the spleen

With the child sitting, the manipulator holds the child's left hand with one hand, and applies rotary pushing with the other hand to the ventral aspect of the child's thumb (fig. 5). The manipulation is repeated for about one minute, and then applied to the right hand.

(6) Point-pressing of the main tendon

With the child sitting, the manipulator holds the child's right hand with one hand and applies point-pressing with the thumb of the other hand to the anterior aspect of the

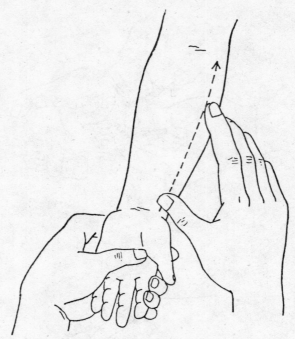

Fig. 3

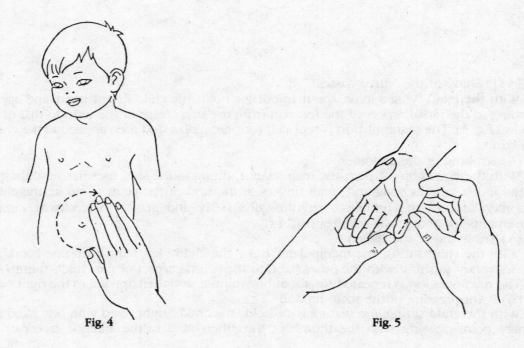

Fig. 4

Fig. 5

164

forearm at the midpoint of the skin crease of the wrist for about thirty seconds (fig. 6). Then similar manipulation is applied to the child's left hand.

NB:

(1) Acupoint massage once a day for 5-7 days may alleviate or cure the night crying.

(2) Regular feeding is recommended. Overfeeding is apt to cause injury to the spleen and stomach. Intake of air while feeding with milk should be prevented.

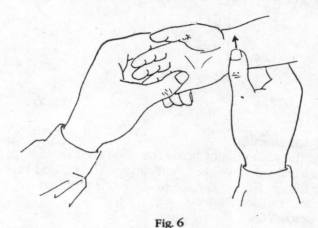

Fig. 6

# Vomiting in Children

Cause: Vomiting is a common symptom in children's diseases, particularly in the diseases of infants. Discussed in this section is only the vomiting due to functional disorders of the gastrointestinal tract, overfeeding with milk, impairment of the stomach by raw, cold, greasy and unsanitary food, or due to improper feeding or crying after suckling.

Main Symptoms: Vomiting soon after eating or immediately after eating, particularly if the intake is somewhat in excess; vomiting on and off with watery vomitus containing undigested milk or food residue, sour and foul in odour, and may be accompanied by abdominal distension which will be relieved after vomiting.

Acupoint Massage: It has the effect of invigorating the spleen, regulating the stomach function and arresting vomiting.

[Manipulation]

(1) Tonifying of the spleen

With the child sitting, the manipulator holds the child's left hand with one hand, places the other hand on the ventral or lateral aspect of the child's thumb, and pushes straight from the tip to the root of the thumb (fig. 1). The manipulation is repeated for about one minute, and then applied to the right thumb.

(2) Kneading of the thenar prominence

With the child sitting, the manipulator holds the child's left hand with one hand, places the other hand on the thenar prominence, and kneads in clockwise direction for about one minute (fig. 2). Then the manipulation is applied to the right thenar prominence in a similar way.

165

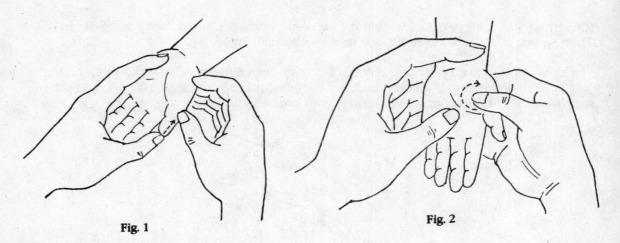

Fig. 1                    Fig. 2

(3) Cleaning of the large intestine

With the child sitting, the manipulator holds the child's left hand with one hand, places the other hand on the radial aspect of the child's index finger, and pushes straight from the root to the tip of the finger (fig. 3). The manipulation is repeated for about one minute, and then applied to the right index finger.

(4) Stroking of Zhongwan (CV 12)

With the child lying supine, the manipulator supports the lateral aspect of the child's abdomen with one hand, and strokes the child's abdomen with the other hand at Zhongwan (CV 12), 4 fingers' breadth superior to the umbilicus, in clockwise circular movements for about two minutes (fig. 4).

(5) Pinching along the spine

With the child lying prone with the back naked to the lower border of the coccyx, the manipulator, bending the fingers naturally and propping the index and middle fingers on the child's coccyx, pushes the right and left hand alternately forward along the spine up to the seventh thoracic vertebra while pinching with the thumb and the index finger,

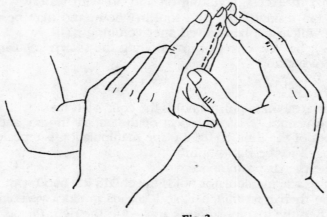

Fig. 3

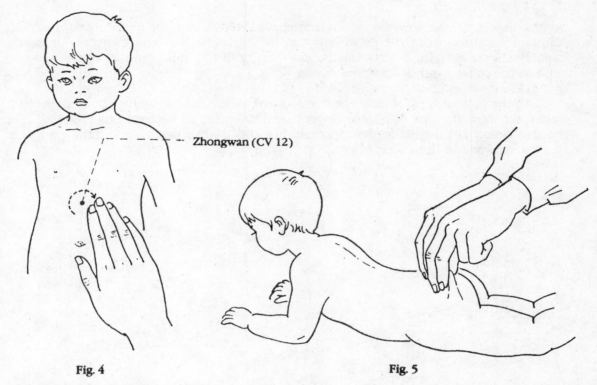

Zhongwan (CV 12)

Fig. 4                                         Fig. 5

gently lifting up the skin once after three pushes and pinches (fig. 5). The manipulation is repeated three times. It is desirable to induce mild redness of the skin along the spine.

NB:

(1) Acupoint massage once daily in mild cases and 2-3 times a day in severe cases usually brings improvement in 3-5 days.

(2) Rational feeding and restriction of greasy or cold foods are recommended.

## Myopia in Teen-agers

Cause: Myopia in teen-agers is chiefly due to improper use of vision, such as dim lighting while reading, reading a book printed in small letters for a long time, reading while riding in a car, or reading while lying, which leads to ametropia. In addition, genetic factors, overfatigue and insufficient sleep may also play a role in the development of myopia.

Main Symptoms: Blurred distant vision with liability of the eyes to be tired and aching and distension of the eyes after reading or writing, headaches and dizziness.

Acupoint Massage: This massage has the effect of promoting blood circulation in the meridians and collaterals and improving eyesight.

[Manipulation]

1. Massage performed by a family member

(1) Pushing of the orbits

With the patient lying supine, the manipulator, sitting behind, applies pushing with the

167

ventral aspect of the thumbs or the index and middle fingers to the patient's orbits, repeatedly starting from the point between the eyebrows and going laterally along the eyebrows separately for three minutes, and then from the inner canthus along the lower orbit to the outer canthus for three minutes (fig. 1).

(2) Point-pressing of Jingming (BL 1)

With the patient lying supine, the manipulator, sitting behind, applies point-pressing of light force with the tips of middle fingers simultaneously to bilateral Jingming (BL 1) in the depression just medial to the inner canthus (fig. 2). It is desirable to induce a feeling of local aching and distension.

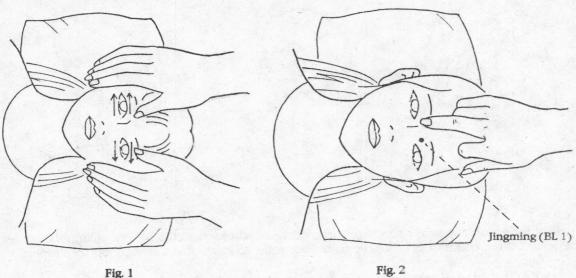

Jingming (BL 1)

Fig. 1                                        Fig. 2

(3) Point-pressing of Xinshu (BL 15) and Ganshu (BL 18)

With the patient taking a sitting position, the manipulator applies point-pressing with the thumb tips simultaneously to bilateral Xinshu (BL 15), 1.5 *cun* lateral to the midpoint between the spinous processes of the fifth and sixth thoracic vertebrae, and Ganshu (BL 18), 1.5 *cun* lateral to the midpoint between the spinous processes of the ninth and tenth thoracic vertebrae, each for one minute (fig. 3). It is desirable to induce a feeling of local aching and distension.

(4) Rubbing of the scalp

With the patient taking a sitting position, the manipulator, standing behind with the fingers slightly bent, rubs and taps the patient's scalp with the fingertips rapidly for about two minutes (fig. 4).

*2. Self-massage*

(1) Stroking of the face

Take a sitting position. Rub the palms warm, then stroke the face with the palms beside the nose, around the orbits, along the forehead and near the ears in clockwise circular movements for about two minutes, and finally move around the eyes for about one minute (fig. 5).

168

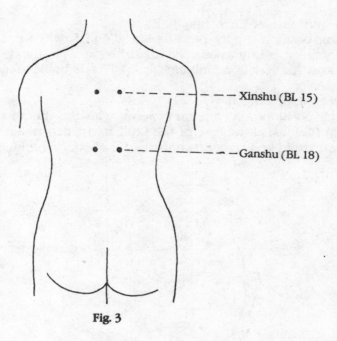

Fig. 3

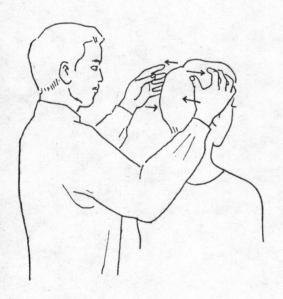

Fig. 4

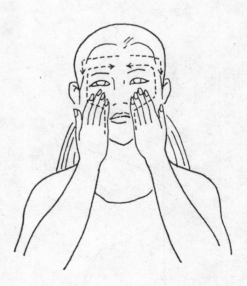

Fig. 5

(2) Pressing-kneading of Cuanzhu (BL 2)

Take a sitting position. Apply pressing-kneading of light force with the tips of the middle fingers simultaneously to bilateral Cuanzhu (BL 2) in the depression at the medial end of the eyebrow for about one minute (fig. 6). It is desirable to induce a feeling of local aching and distension.

(3) Point-pressing of Fengchi (GB 20)

Take a sitting position. Apply point-pressing with the thumb tips simultaneously to bilateral Fengchi (GB 20) at the base of the skull, in the depression between the heads of the sternocleidomastoid and trapezius muscles, for about one minute (fig. 7).

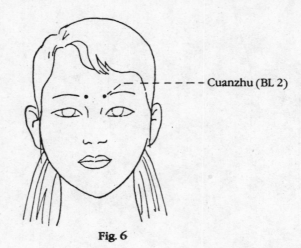

Cuanzhu (BL 2)

Fig. 6

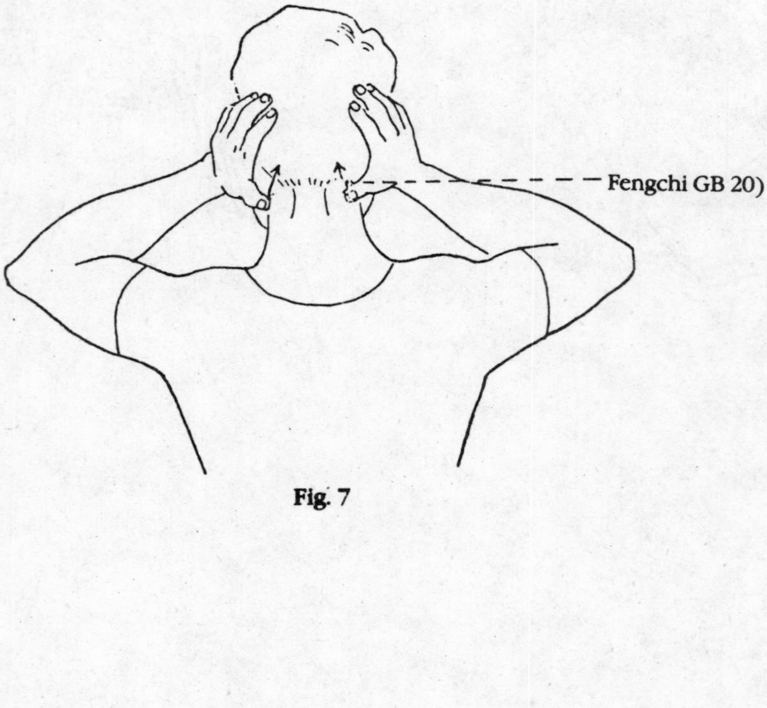

Fengchi GB 20)

Fig. 7

(4) Pressing-kneading of Jianjing (GB 21)

Take a sitting position. Crossing the hands, apply pressing-kneading with the tips of the middle fingers simultaueously to Jianjing (GB 21) of the opposite side for about two minutes. Jianjing (GB 21) is located at the midpoint of the line joining the spinous process of the seventh thoracic vertebra and the acromion (fig. 8).

NB:

(1) It is advised to perform this acupoint massage 1-2 times a day. The manipulation should be soft and gentle with concentration of the mind and avoidance of touching the eyeball.

(2) Physical exercise and correction of habits harmful to the vision are recommended.

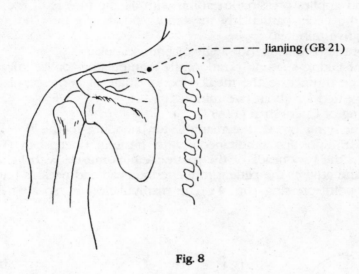

Fig. 8

# IV. Orthopedic Diseases

## Stiff Necks

Cause: Stiff necks are usually found when getting up in the morning. They often occur in those with weak constitution and overfatigue who take an unfavorable position during sleep, having the pillow too high, too low or too hard, which causes overextension, twisting or strain of a group of cervical muscles. Furthermore, exposure to cold leads to stagnation of *qi* and blood in the muscles, meridians and collaterals, resulting in spasm and pain.

Main Symptoms: Aching, spasm and rigidity of one side of the neck, often accompanied by deviation of the head to the affected side and difficulty in turning the head, and even radiating pain to the shoulder and back of the affected side. Muscular spasm with marked tenderness and palpable cord-like mass and limitation in motion of the neck on examination.

Acupoint Massage: This massage has the effect of soothing the muscles, promoting blood circulation, relieving spasm and arresting pain.

## [Manipulation]

*1. Massage performed by a family member*

(1) Pressing of Fengfu (GV 16), Fengmen (BL 12) and Tianzong (SI 11)

With the patient taking a sitting position, the manipulator, standing behind, applies pressing with the thumb tip to Fengfu (GV 16) on the posterior midline of the neck, in the depression just inferior to the occipital protuberance and 1 *cun* superior to the hairline, Fengmen (BL 12), 1.5 *cun* lateral to the midpoint between the second and third thoracic vertebrae, and Tianzong (SI 11) on the posterior aspect of the shoulder, in the centre of the infraspinous fossa, each for about one minute (fig. 1).

(2) Pressing-kneading of the neck

With the patient taking a sitting position, the manipulator supports the patient's head with one hand, and applies pressing-kneading with all the fingers of the other hand to lateral aspects of the neck, particularly the tender points (fig. 2). The manipulation is repeated for about five minutes.

(3) Kneading of the mediosuperior angle of both scapulae

With the patient taking a sitting position, the manipulator applies kneading with the ventral aspect of the thumbs to the mediosuperior angle of both scapulae (fig. 3). The manipulation is repeated for about two minutes.

(4) Point-pressing of Chengshan (BL 57)

With the patient lying prone, the manipulator, standing to the side, applies point-pressing with the thumb tips simultaneously to bilateral Chengshan (BL 57) in the depression between the two heads of the gastrocnemius muscle with light force at first and then heavier, and advises the patient to move the head and neck as much as possible while performing point-pressing (fig. 4). The manipulation is repeated for about one minute.

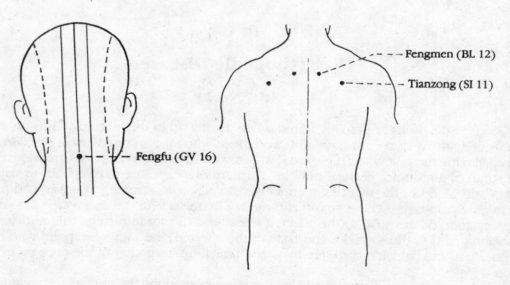

Fengmen (BL 12)

Tianzong (SI 11)

Fengfu (GV 16)

Fig. 1

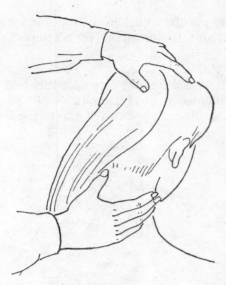

**Fig. 2**

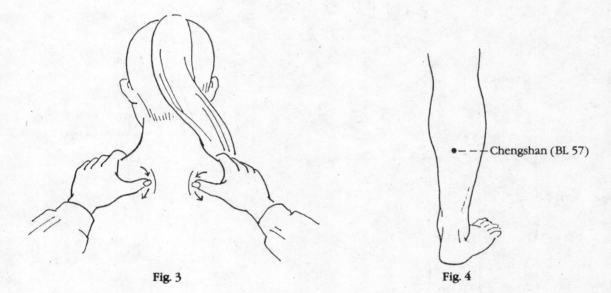

**Fig. 3**

Chengshan (BL 57)

**Fig. 4**

*2. Self-massage*
(1) Pressing-kneading of Fengchi (GB 20)
Take a sitting position. Placing the thumb on Fengchi (GB 20) at the base of the skull, in the depression inferior to the occipital protuberance, and supporting the occiput with the other four fingers, apply pressing-kneading with force for about two minutes (fig. 5).
(2) Kneading-grasping of Jianjing (GB 21) of the affected side
Take a sitting position. Apply kneading and grasping with the thumb, index and middle

173

fingers to Jianjing (GB 21) at the midpoint of the line joining the spinous process of the seventh thoracic vertebra and the acromion (fig. 6). Repeat the manipulation for about two minutes.

(3) Point-pressing of Zusanli (ST 36)

Take a sitting position with the upper trunk slightly bent forward. Apply point-pressing with the thumb tips simultaneously to bilateral Zusanli (ST 36), 3 *cun* inferior to the lateral aspect of the knee and one finger's breadth lateral to the tibial crest for about one minute (fig. 7).

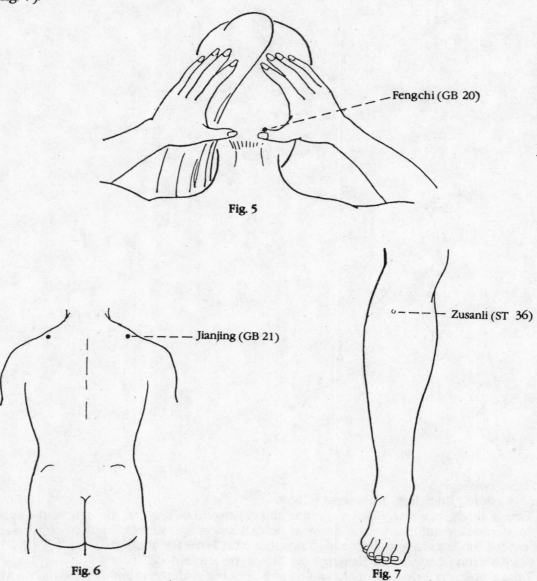

Fengchi (GB 20)

Fig. 5

Jianjing (GB 21)

Zusanli (ST 36)

Fig. 6

Fig. 7

NB:

(1) Stiff necks can be cured by performing acupoint massage once a day for 2-3 days. Even if it has already lasted for a long time, good effect can still be obtained after several times of massage.

(2) It is recommended to use a pillow of appropriate height and avoid exposure of the neck to cold so as to prevent recurrence.

## Cervical Spondylosis

Cause: Cervical spondylosis is a syndrome characterized by pressure or stimulation of the cervical nerves due to various factors, commonly occurring in the aged. Injuries and degenerative changes of the cervical vertebrae play an important role in the pathogenesis of cervical spondylosis. Various acute and chronic traumatic injuries may cause damage to the intervertebral discs, ligaments and posterior joint capsules, resulting in this syndrome.

In case of degenerative changes of the cervical intervertebral discs, water in the vertebrae is gradually absorbed, and the intervertebral discs become thinner, with narrowing of the intervertebral space and laxation of perivertebral ligaments and joint capsules, so that the stability of cervical spine is impaired and its motion increased, leading to hyperosteogeny and calcification of the ligaments with pressure or stimulation on cervical nerves, cervical spinal cord or main blood vessels of the neck, and hence cervical spondylosis.

Main Symptoms: Intermittent or persistent discomfort or pain of the neck at the onset, gradually worsening along with development of pathological changes, radiating pain and numbness of the neck, shoulders, back, chest and upper limbs, with aggravation of pain during coughing, sneezing, exertion of force on defecation, bending or moving the head. If the spinal cord is pressed, there is numbness and weakness of the limbs, tremoring of the arms, limitation in motion and even paralysis. If the sympathetic nerve is pressed, dizziness, migraine, headaches, a sensation of suffocation in the chest and coldness of the limbs develop. X-ray examination is of significance for the diagnosis.

Acupoint Massage: This massage has the effect of improving blood circulation of the neck, relieving spasm and pain, eliminating swelling, dissolving adhesion and alleviating the pressure on the nerve root.

[Manipulation]

1. Massage performed by a family member

(1) Kneading-pinching of the neck, upper back and affected limb

With the patient taking a sitting position, the manipulator, standing behind, supports the patient's head with one hand, and applies kneading and pinching with the other hand to both sides of the neck up and down for about two minutes, then to the shoulders, upper back and affected upper limb for about three minutes (fig. 1).

(2) Pressing-kneading of Jianjing (GB 21), Jianyu (LI 15), Quchi (LI 11) and Hegu (LI 4)

With the patient taking a sitting position, the manipulator, standing to the side, applies pressing and kneading with the right and left thumb alternately to Jianjing (GB 21) at the midpoint of the line joining the spinous process of the seventh thoracic vertebra and the acromion, Jianyu (LI 15) in the centre of the depression at the end of the shoulder as the

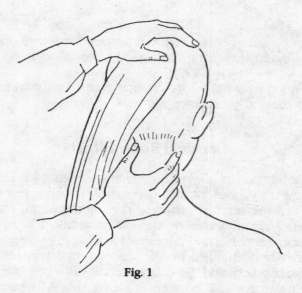

**Fig. 1**

arm is in full abduction, Quchi (LI 11) in the depression at the lateral end of the elbow crease as the elbow is flexed, and Hegu (LI 4) between the first and second metacarpal bones and on the radial aspect of the second metacarpal, each for one minute (fig. 2).

(3) Traction of the affected limb

With the patient taking a sitting position, the manipulator, standing to the side, holds the patient's upper arm with one hand from behind, lifting it somewhat upward and outward, and holds the distal end of the patient's forearm with the other hand, pulling

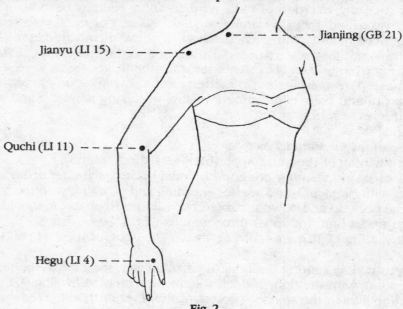

**Fig. 2**

downward and then relaxing (fig. 3). The manipulation is repeated for about one minute.

(4) Poking of the tender points

With the patient taking a sitting position, the manipulator, standing to the side, holds the patient's shoulder with one hand, and applies, with the thumb tip of the other hand, poking upward, downward, rightward and leftward each for 3-5 times to the tender points on the neck, shoulders and back while the patient is actively moving the head and neck to the right and left (fig. 4).

(5) Scrubbing of the affected limb

With the patient taking a sitting position with the affected limb relaxed, the manipulator, standing to the side, scrubs the limb with palms from the shoulder along the upper arm to the distal end of the forearm (fig. 5). The manipulation is repeated 5-7 times.

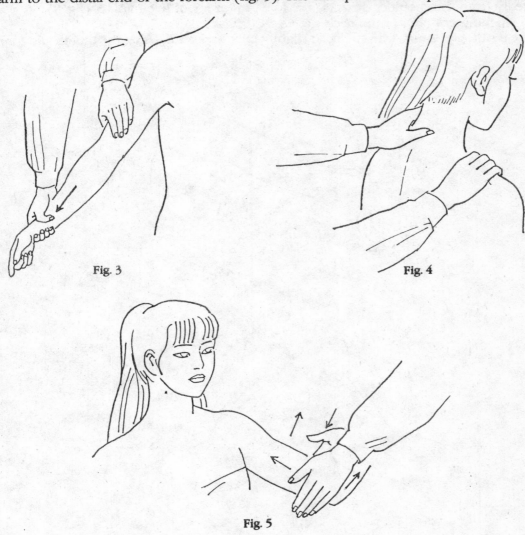

Fig. 3

Fig. 4

Fig. 5

(6) Vibrating of the affected limb

With the patient lying supine with the affected limb relaxed, the manipulator, standing to the side and holding the distal end of the affected limb, makes slow vibrations like waves to soothe the muscles and joints (fig. 6). The manipulation is repeated 5-7 times.

2. *Self-massage*

(1) Pressing-kneading of Fengchi (GB 20)

Take a sitting position. Placing the thumb tips at Fengchi (GB 20) in the depression inferior to the occipital protuberance, apply kneading repeatedly for about one minute (fig. 7)

(2) Rubbing of the affected limb

Take a sitting position. Using the palm of the healthy side, rub the affected limb repeatedly from the shoulder down to the forearm for about five minutes (fig. 8)

(3) Pinching-grasping of the neck

Take a sitting position with the head slightly bent backward. Using the thumb and four

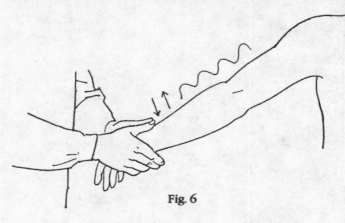

Fig. 6

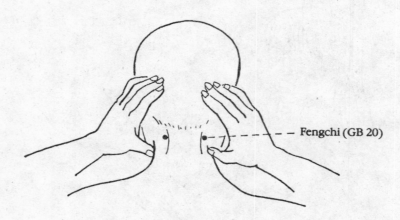

Fengchi (GB 20)

Fig. 7

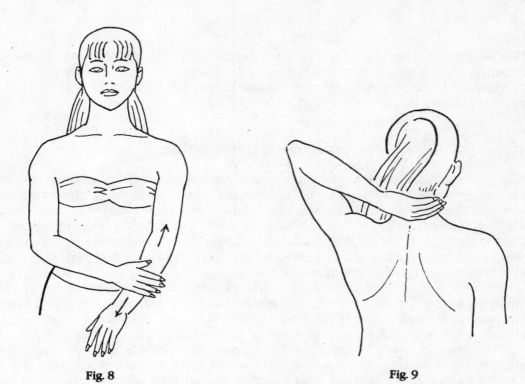

Fig. 8                                                    Fig. 9

fingers of the hand of the healthy side to pinch and grasp the neck from the upper to the lower (fig. 9). Repeat the manipulation for about three minutes.

(4) Point-pressing of Jianwaishu (SI 14)

Take a sitting position. Apply point-pressing with the tip of the middle finger of the healthy side to Jianwaishu (SI 14), 3 *cun* lateral to the midpoint between the spinous processes of the first and second thoracic vertebrae, for about three minutes (fig. 10).

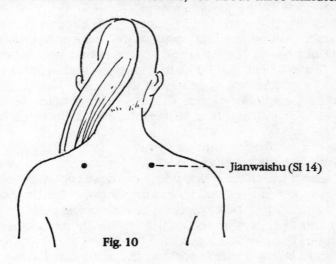

— Jianwaishu (SI 14)

Fig. 10

NB:

(1) It is advised to perform this acupoint massage once a day or every other day. The manipulation should be soft and even with no violent actions.

(2) Exercise of the neck with flexion, extension and circular motions is necessary for the treatment of the current disease and prevention of recurrence.

# Periarthritis of the Shoulder

Cause: Periarthritis of the shoulder is a degenerative and inflammatory lesion of the joint capsule and surrounding soft tissues of the shoulder, often occurring in those over fifty years of age. The motion of shoulder joint is frequent in daily life and work, so that the surrounding tissues are apt to suffer from acute or chronic strain by rubbing and squeezing from various sources. If the injured shoulder is not well treated in due time, or the patient neglects the necessary exercise of the injured shoulder despite of the pain, and if the shoulder is exposed to cold, periarthritis may occur.

According to traditional Chinese medicine, insufficiency of *qi* and blood to nourish the local muscles in the aged is the chief endogenous cause of periarthritis of the shoulder, while exposure to wind, cold and damp as well as strain is the exogenous cause.

Main Symptoms: At the early stage there is pain of the shoulder with limitation in motion, sometimes involving the neck, back and upper limb. The pain is usually aggravated at night, disturbing the sleep, but becomes better after getting up and taking mild exercises. Later on the motion of the affected limb is further limited with difficulty in dressing and undressing, combing the hair, and lifting the arm. In a chronic case, there may be muscular atrophy of the shoulder.

Acupoint Massage: This massage has the effect of removing obstruction from the meridians and collaterals, promoting blood circulation, arresting pain, soothing the joints and loosening the adhesions.

[Manipulation]

*1. Massage performed by a family member*

(1) Point-pressing of Jianyu (LI 15), Jianjing (GB 21) and Tianzong (SI 11)

With the patient taking a sitting position, the manipulator, standing to the side, holds the patient's shoulder with one hand and applies point-pressing with the thumb tip of the other hand to bilateral Jianyu (LI 15), in the depression anterior to the shoulder joint at the inferior border of acromial extremity of the clavicle, Jianjing (GB 21), at the midpoint of the line joining the spinous process of the seventh thoracic vertebra and the acromion, and Tianzong (SI 11), in the centre of the infraspinous fossa, each for about one minute (fig. 1).

(2) Pushing of the affected limb

With the patient taking a sitting position, the manipulator, standing to the side and lifting the forearm of the effected side with one hand, applies pushing with the other palm along the lateral aspect of the forearm and the elbow to the shoulder and back repeatedly for about two minutes, and then, changing hands, applies pushing along the medial aspect of the forearm and the elbow to the armpit repeatedly for another two minutes (fig. 2).

(3) Kneading of the affected shoulder

With the patient taking a sitting position, the manipulator holds and repeatedly kneads

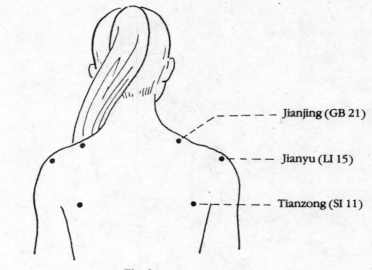

Jianjing (GB 21)

Jianyu (LI 15)

Tianzong (SI 11)

Fig. 1

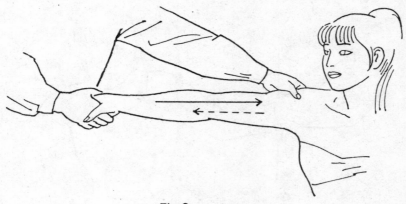

Fig. 2

the affected shoulder for about five minutes (fig. 3).

(4) Poking of the tender points

With the patient taking a sitting position, the manipulator, standing to the side, pokes the tender points of the patient's shoulder with one hand, and at the same time makes flexing, extending and circular movements of the affected limb with the other hand for about one minute (fig. 4).

(5) Shaking and pulling of the affected limb

With the patient lying prone with the muscles of the affected limb relaxed, the manipulator, standing to the side and holding the wrist of the affected limb with both hands, gradually pulls it and at the same time shakes it slowly and evenly to cause wave-like movements (fig. 5). The manipulation is repeated for one minute.

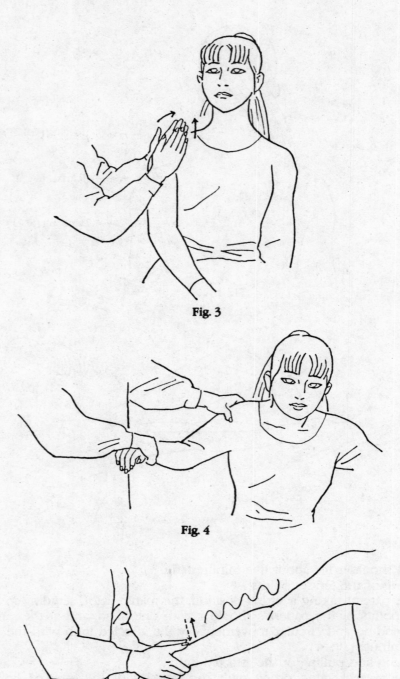

Fig. 3

Fig. 4

Fig. 5

182

### 2. Self-massage

(1) Pressing-kneading of the affected shoulder

Take a sitting position. Placing the palm of the healthy side closely against the affected shoulder, press and at the same time knead it around the acromion in combination with active rotatory movements of the affected shoulder (fig. 6). The manipulation is repeated for about five minutes.

(2) Patting of the affected shoulder

Take a sitting position. Half clenching the hand of the healthy side into a fist, pat the affected shoulder with the palmar aspect of the fist rhythmically for one minute (fig. 7).

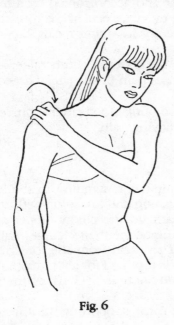

Fig. 6

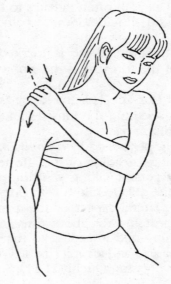

Fig. 7

(3) Swinging of the arm

Take a standing position with the feet apart and the back slightly bent over. Placing the healthy arm on the waist, swing the affected arm in circular movements with gradually increasing amplitude and speed. The exercise is performed for five minutes each time.

NB:

(1) During massage treatment, the affected shoulder should be protected from cold.

(2) At the early stage of periarthritis of the shoulder when the inflammation is accompanied with severe local pain, the manipulation should be soft and gentle.

## External Humeral Epicondylitis

Cause: External humeral epicondylitis, also called tennis elbow, often occurs in carpenters, construction workers, fitters, tennis, table tennis and badminton players and housewives. The external humeral epicondyle is the place where the extensor muscle tendons, such as long radial extensor muscle of wrist, short radial extensor muscle of wrist, common extensor muscle of fingers and ulnar extensor muscle of wrist attach. Prone motion of the forearm as one is falling down on the ground, turning the elbow with force, repeated exertion of force with the wrist too violently or too long, carrying a weight for a long time or throwing a heavy thing may cause overtraction of the extensor muscles. resulting in external humeral epicondylitis with rigidity, pain and functional disturbance of the elbow joint.

Main Symptoms: At the onset there is occasional pain in the lateral aspect of the elbow, gradually increasing in severity and becoming persistent. The pain is aggravated by carrying things, twisting a towel or sweeping the floor and accompanied by a feeling of distension. The pain often radiates to the extensor and radial aspects of the forearm, wrist, upper arm and shoulder. Severe pain may cause difficulty in taking meals, dressing and sleeping.

On examination, there is marked tenderness at the external humeral epicondyle. Pronation of the forearm as the elbow is extended causes pain in the lateral aspect of the elbow.

Acupoint Massage: This massage has the effect of promoting blood circulation, removing blood stasis, soothing the muscles and tendons and relieving pain.

**[Manipulation]**

*1. Massage performed by a family member*

(1) Pushing-kneading of the affected limb

With the patient taking a sitting position, the manipulator, standing to the side and supporting the affected limb with one hand, applies pushing and kneading with the other hand to the lateral aspect of the arm from the forearm to the elbow, upper arm and shoulder repeatedly for about three minutes. The manipulator then changes hands and applies pushing and kneading to the medial aspect of the arm from the forearm to the elbow, upper arm and armpit (fig. 1). The manipulation is repeated for about three minutes.

(2) Point-pressing Quchi (LI 11), Shaohai (HT 3) and Shousanli (LI 10) of the affected limb

With the patient taking a sitting position, the manipulator, supporting the affected limb with one hand, applies point-pressing with the thumb tip of the other hand to Quchi (LI 11), in the depression at the lateral end of the elbow crease as the elbow is flexed, Shaohai (HT 3), on the ulnar aspect of the elbow, at the end of the elbow crease as the elbow is flexed, and Shousanli (LI 10), 2 *cun* inferior to the depression at the lateral end of the elbow crease as the elbow is flexed, each for about one minute (fig. 2).

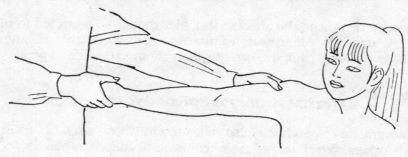

Fig. 1

184

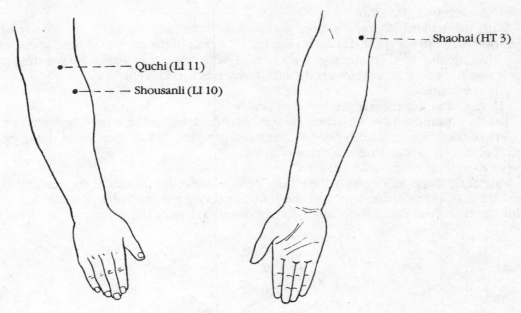

Quchi (LI 11)

Shousanli (LI 10)

Shaohai (HT 3)

**Fig. 2**

(3) Pressing-kneading of the tender point at the external humeral epicondyle

With the patient taking a sitting position, the manipulator, standing to the side and holding with one hand the wrist of the patient's affected limb with the palm facing upward and the elbow with the other hand, places the thumb on the lateral aspect of the elbow and makes the elbow flex and extend, at the same time applying pressing-kneading to and fro with the thumb perpendicular to the tender point at the external humeral epicondyle for about three minutes (fig. 3). The manipulation should be performed with appropriate force, and it is desirable to induce a feeling of aching and distension.

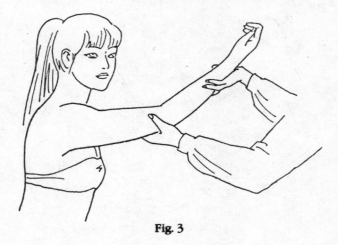

**Fig. 3**

(4) Swaying of the elbow

With the patient taking a sitting position, the manipulator, fixing the affected elbow with one hand, placing the thumb on the lateral aspect of the external humeral epicondyle, and holding the forearm in slight abduction with the other hand, sways the forearm clockwise for thirty seconds with the elbow joint as the axis (fig. 4).

2. *Self-massage*

(1) Pinching-grasping of the affected limb

Take a sitting position with the elbow slightly bent. Using the thumb, index and middle fingers of the healthy side, apply pinching and grasping to the muscles of the upper arm and forearm for about three minutes (fig. 5).

(2) Kneading of the affected area

Take a sitting position with the elbow bent. Placing the thumb of the healthy side on the lateral aspect of the elbow and the four fingers on the medial aspect, apply kneading with the thumb to the affected area for about two minutes (fig. 6).

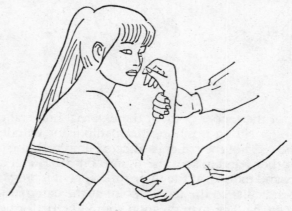

**Fig. 4**

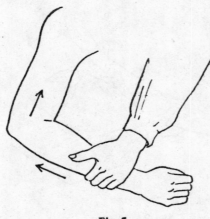

**Fig. 5**

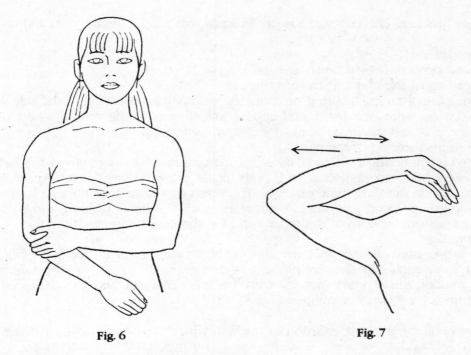

**Fig. 6**

**Fig. 7**

(3) Flexing and extending of the elbow

Take a sitting position with the elbow slightly bent. Placing the palm of the healthy side on the olecranon of the affected elbow, apply pressing to the tender point 6f the external humeral epicondyle while flexing and extending the elbow actively for about two minutes (fig. 7).

NB:

(1) During the massage treatment, appropriate rest of the affected limb is necessary, otherwise the therapeutic effect will not be satisfactory and the epicondylitis will be liable to recur.

(2) The affected elbow should be kept warm.

## Thecal Cyst on the Dorsum of the Wrist

Cause: The etiology of thecal cyst on the dorsum of the wrist is not clear. It is generally realized that the formation of thecal cysts is related to degenerative changes of the joint capsule, ligaments and tendon sheath, denaturation of the mucus in the joint capsule, acute or chronic trauma and protrusion of joint capsule or tendon sheath. The thecal cyst often occurs in young people, particularly in women.

Main Symptoms: The cyst is spherical in shape with a smooth surface and a clear-cut border but no adhesion with the skin. It grows slowly. On palpitation it gives a cystic feeling at the onset, but gradually it becomes smaller and harder. It sticks out more evidently when the wrist is flexed to the palmar side. Usually is causes no symptoms, but in some cases it may produce a feeling of aching, distension and weakness.

187

Acupoint Massage: This massage has the effect of removing the stagnation and nodulation.

**[Manipulation]**

*1. Massage performed by a family member*

(1) Kneading of the cyst and its surroundings

With the patient taking a sitting position, the manipulator, standing to the side, holds the affected wrist with one hand, and applies kneading with the ventral aspect of the thumb to the cyst and its surroundings for three minutes (fig. 1).

(2) Pressing-squeezing of the cyst

With the patient taking a sitting position, the manipulator, standing in front and holding the distal end of the affected wrist with both hands, pulls the wrist and flexes it to the palmar side, and at the same time places both thumbs on the sides of the cyst to break it by squeezing and pressing. Then hold the forearm with one hand, pressing and kneading the cyst area with the thumb of the other hand for about five minutes (fig. 2).

*2. Self-massage*

Take a sitting position and place the affected limb on a table with the hand flexed to the palmar side. Break the cyst by pressing with the thumb of the healthy side while repeatedly making active rotary motions with the wrist. Then rub and knead the cyst and its surroundings for about five minutes (fig. 3).

NB:

(1) After breaking the cyst, exertion of strength with the wrist should be avoided. It is necessary to knead the cyst area 5-7 minutes daily for prevention of recurrence.

(2) Wet and hot dressing is recommended.

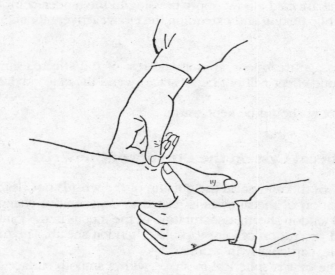

**Fig. 1**

188

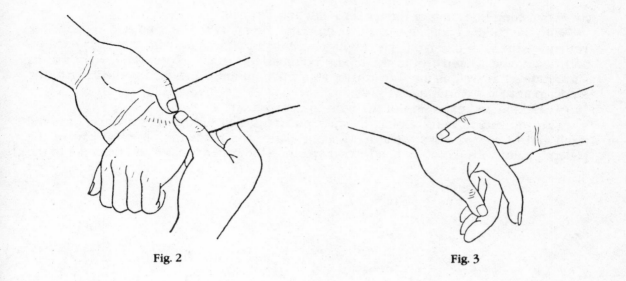

Fig. 2            Fig. 3

## Stenosing Tenovaginitis at the Styloid Process of the Radius

Cause: Stenosing tenovaginitis at the styloid process of the radius is due to constant extreme flexion of the wrist to the radial side, acute sprain and chronic strain, as occurring in laundry workers, packing workers, knitting workers, shoemakers, and those who frequently hold a baby in their arms or cut up meat and vegetables. All these actions may cause traumatic inflammation, edema and thickening of the tendon and stenosis of the tendon sheath. The disease may occur at any age, but more frequently in women.

Main Symptoms: Pain of wrist, gradually aggravated, usually localized at the styloid process of the radius, but sometimes radiating to the hand and forearm. Reduced grip strength, subcutaneous bean-like masses palpable at the styloid process of the radius along with marked tenderness, limitation in motion of the wrist and thumb, aggravation of the pain during adduction of the thumb, clenching of the fist, and flexion of the wrist to the ulnar aspect.

Acupoint Massage: This massage has the effect of activating blood circulation, removing blood stasis, promoting the subsidence of swelling and relieving pain.

**[Manipulation]**

*1. Massage performed by a family member*

(1) Pressing of Hegu (LI 4), Waiguan(TE 5) and Shousanli (LI 10)

With the patient lying supine, the manipulator, sitting by the affected side, supports the the patient's forearm with one hand, and applies pressing with the thumb of the other hand to Hegu (LI 4), between the first and second metacarpal bones and on the radial aspect of the second metacarpal, Waiguan (TE 5), on the dorsum of the forearm, 2 *cun* superior to the transverse wrist crease between the radius and ulna, and Shousanli (LI 10) on the radial aspect of the forearm, 2 *cun* inferior to the lateral end of the elbow crease as the elbow is flexed, each for one minute (fig. 1).

(2) Pushing-kneading of the tender point and forearm

With the patient lying supine, the manipulator, sitting by the affected side, supports the patient's wrist with one hand, and applies pushing and kneading with the other hand up and down, and to and fro, to the tender point on the radial aspect of the wrist and its surroundings as well as the forearm for about five minutes, and then particularly to the tender point for two minutes (fig. 2).

(3) Flexion and extension of the wrist under traction

With the patient lying supine, the manipulator, sitting by the affected side, fixes the distal end of the patient's forearm with one hand, and holds the proximal part of the patient's palm with the other hand, slowly rotating the patient's hand and flexing it to the

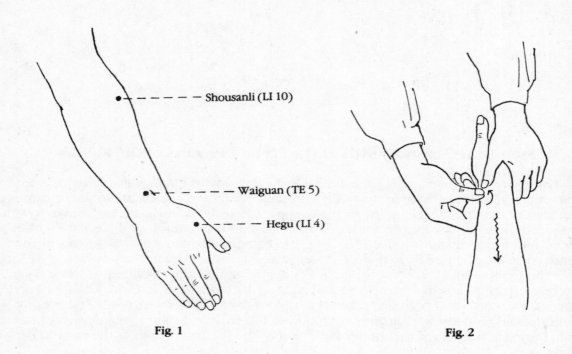

| Fig. 1 | Fig. 2 |

palmar side, extending it to the dorsal side and deviating it to the ulnar side while pulling the wrist with light force (fig. 3). The manipulation is repeated 5-7 times.

(4) Stretching of the thumb of the affected limb

With the patient lying supine, the manipulator, fixing the distal end of the patient's forearm, and pressing the proximal end of the patient's thumb from both sides with the index and middle fingers in a flexed position, stretches the thumb with force by the two hands for about one minute, and then makes passive adduction and abduction of the thumb while stretching for about one minute (fig. 4).

2. Self-massage

(1) Grasping-pinching of the forearm

Take a sitting position, placing the affected limb on a table. Apply grasping and pinching

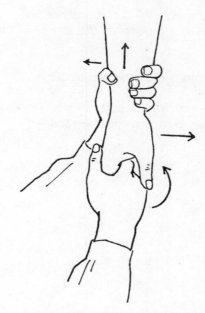

**Fig. 3**

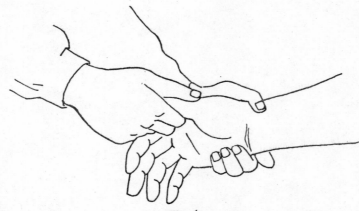

**Fig. 4**

with the thumb and the other four fingers of the healthy hand to the forearm from the elbow to the wrist (fig. 5). Repeat the manipulation for about two minutes.

(2) Rubbing-kneading of the affected area

Take a sitting position, placing the affected limb on a table. Apply rubbing and kneading with the ventral aspect of the thumb of the healthy side to the forearm from the middle portion of the radial aspect of the forearm to the wrist (fig. 6). Repeat the manipulation for about three minutes.

(3) Rubbing of the ulnar aspect of the forearm

Take a sitting position with the affected limb bent and placed in front of the chest.

Apply rubbing with the ventral aspect of the thumb of the healthy side to the forearm from the upper border of the styloid process of the radius to the wrist (fig. 7). Repeat the rubbing for one minute.

NB:

(1) Excessive flexion and extension of the wrist and fingers should be avoided during the massage.

(2) All the factors that may precipitate pain should be avoided; wet hot dressing or application of plasters to alleviate pain is recommended.

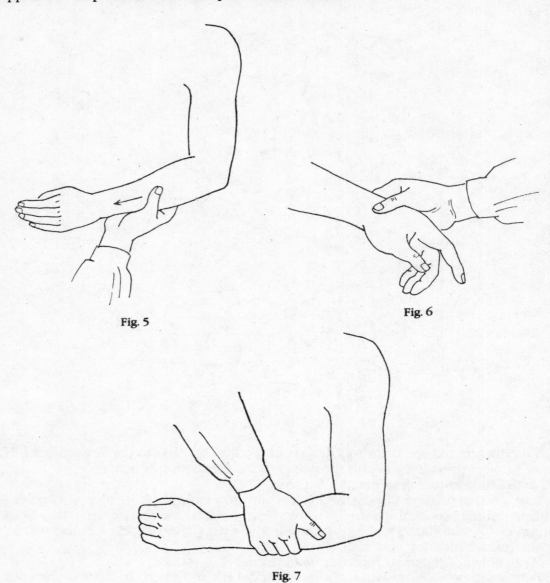

Fig. 5

Fig. 6

Fig. 7

# Acute Lumbar Sprain

Cause: Acute lumbar sprain refers to sprain and contusion of the soft tissue in the lumbar region, particularly in the lumbo-sacral region, sacroiliac articulation and sacrospinal muscle. It is often due to sudden twist of the waist, overstretching of the lumbo-sacral muscles, ligaments, articulations and synovium when carrying a thing too heavy for the muscles, harmful posture during strenuous exercise, falling down on the ground or picking up a thing from the ground, coughing, sneezing or a direct stroke at the lower back.

Main Symptoms: After the traumatic injury, pain in the lumbar region, inability to stand upright and walk, difficulty in sitting, lying down and turning over, or even inability to get up. The pain is aggravated by coughing, sneezing and deep breathing. In some cases, the pain is mild immediately after sprain, but gradually becomes worse after half a day or on the next day. On examination there is local muscular tension with marked tenderness.

Acupoint Massage: This massage has the effect of soothing the muscles and ligaments, promoting blood circulation and relieving pain.

[Manipulation]

*1. Manipulation by a family member*

(1) Point-pressing of Shenshu (BL 23), Huantiao (GB 30) and Weizhong (BL 40)

With the patient lying prone, the manipulator applies point-pressing with the thumb tips to Shenshu (BL 23), 1.5 *cun* lateral to the midpoint between the spinous processes of the second and third lumbar vertebrae, Huantiao (GB 30) on the buttocks and in the depression posterior to the greater trochanter when standing, and Weizhong (BL 40) on the posterior aspect of the knee, at the centre of the popliteal skin crease, each for one minute (fig. 1).

(2) Pushing-kneading of the back

With the patient lying prone, the manipulator, standing to the side, applies pushing while kneading with the right and left palm alternately to the back from the upper part to the lumbo-sacral region and from the lumbar region to the upper back along the Bladder Meridian for about five minutes, and then particularly to the lumbo-sacral region until there is a feeling of warmth in the lumbar region (fig. 2). The manipulation is performed with light force at first and then with gradually increased force along as the muscle spasm is relieved.

(3) Pressing of Chengshan (BL 57) with the elbow

With the patient lying prone, the manipulator, standing to the side, holds the patient's shank with one hand and flexes the elbow of the other arm, applying pressing perpendicularly and persistently to Chengshan (BL 57) in the centre of the posterior aspect of the leg (fig. 3). At the same time the manipulator asks the patient to get up, supporting the body with the hands on the bed and repeat coughing while swaying the waist rightward, leftward, upward and backward. After the patient takes the prone position again, the manipulation is repeated 2-3 times. The lower back pain is usually alleviated immediately and the motion of the back improved.

(4) Rubbing-patting of the lumbo-sacral region

The patient takes a squatting position with the heels touching the floor and the upper trunk slightly bent forward. The manipulator, standing to the side, supports the patient's shoulder with one hand, and rubs the lumbo-sacral region with the other palm from the

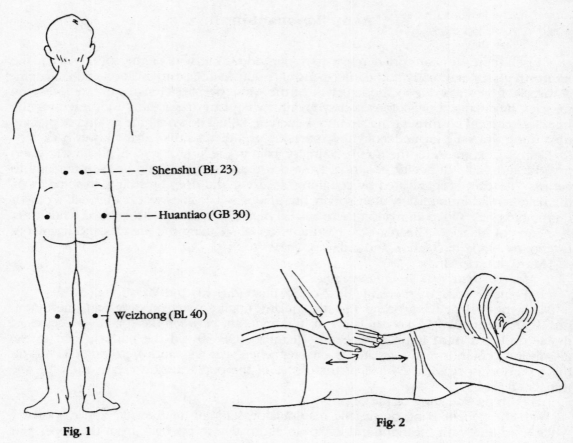

Shenshu (BL 23)

Huantiao (GB 30)

Weizhong (BL 40)

**Fig. 1**

**Fig. 2**

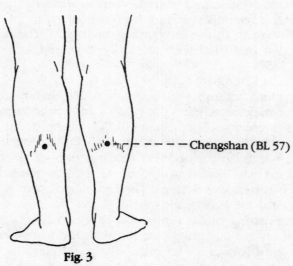

Chengshan (BL 57)

**Fig. 3**

194

upper to the lower until causing warmth in that region, and then closes the fingers together to lightly pat the lumbo-sacral region several times (fig. 4).

*2. Self-massage*

(1) Rotating and swaying of the waist

Stand upright with the feet apart and arms akimbo. Repeatedly rotate and sway the waist from the right to left or vice versa for two minutes (fig. 5).

(2) Kneading of the tender points in the lumbo-sacral region

Take a sitting position and clench the fists. Repeatedly knead and press the tender points of the lumbo-sacral region with the metacarpophalangeal articulation for two minutes (fig. 6).

NB:

(1) Acupoint massage by a family member once daily usually gives good effect for the treatment of acute lumbar sprain.

(2) It is advised to have rest in a hard bed for 5-7 days and keep the lower back warm.

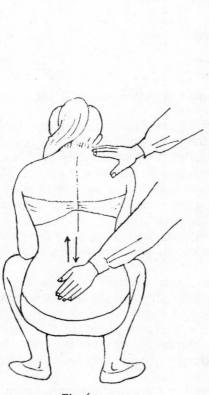

Fig. 4

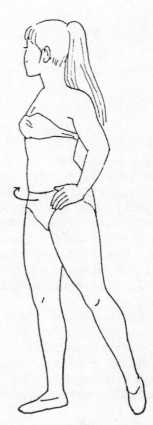

Fig. 5

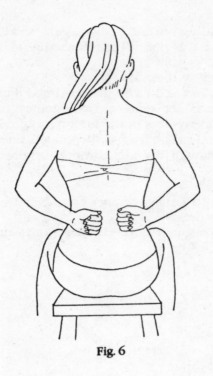

Fig. 6

## Prolapse of the Lumbar Intervertebral Disc

Cause: The internal causes of prolapse of the lumbar intervertebral disc are degenerative changes, atrophy and reduced elasticity of the intervertebral disc and congenital defect. The external cause is traumatic injury of the lower back, particularly lumbar strain such as sudden twisting of the lower back while exertion with the back bent over, lifting a heavy thing or violent physical labor. All these factors may lead to rupture of fibrous rings and protrusion of the pulpiform neucleus, putting pressure on the spinal cord or stimulation on the nerve root, producing pain in the lower back and leg.

In some cases, there is evident history of trauma, and prolapse of the lumbar intervertebral disc occurs after a mere sudden violent cough or sneeze, or due to exposure to cold during sleep.

Main Symptoms: Lower back pain usually with a history of acute lumbar sprain or chronic strain and repeated attacks of the pain after the injury for a period of time. Thereafter, the pain extends from one buttock to a lower limb along the area innervated by the sciatic nerve of one side, including the posterior aspect of the thigh and latero-posterior aspect of the shank and radiating to the lateral aspect of the back of the foot, the heel and toes. The pain is aggravated by coughing, sneezing, defecation and exertion while bending over.

Examination often reveals scoliosis and reduced anterior curvature, and limitation of the spine in motion, more marked during anteflexion. The tender points are usually located

196

at the interspinal space or beside the vertebra between the fourth and fifth lumbar vertebrae or between the fifth lumbar vertebrae and first sacral vertebrae, and pressing on these points can induce or aggravate the radiating pain. Some patients complain of numbness of the posterio-lateral aspect of the shank, back of the foot, heel or sole, and have hypoesthesia.

Acupoint Massage: This massage has the effect of relieving spasm and pain, promoting blood circulation and removing blood stasis.

**[Manipulation]**

*1. Massage performed by a family member*

(1) Pushing of the Bladder Meridian

With the patient lying prone, the manipulator, standing to the side and placing the hands closely against the patient's back, applies pushing with the right and left hand alternately along the Bladder Meridian from the first thoracic vertebra to the lumbo-sacral region, and then to the affected leg from the posterior aspect of the buttock and lateral aspect of the leg to the heel (fig. 1). The massage is repeated for about three minutes with force penetrating deep into the tissue.

(2) Kneading of the back

With the patient lying prone, the manipulator, standing to the side, applies kneading with the right and left palm alternately to the patient's back from the upper to the lumbo-sacral region and then in the reverse direction repeatedly for about three minutes (fig. 2). Then the kneading is applied particularly to the lumbo-sacral region until there is a feeling of warmth and alleviation of pain.

(3) Point-pressing of Huantiao (GB 30), Weizhong (BL 40) and Chengshan (BL 57)

With the patient lying prone, the manipulator applies point-pressing with the thumb tip to Huantiao (GB 30) on the buttock and in the depression posterior to the greater

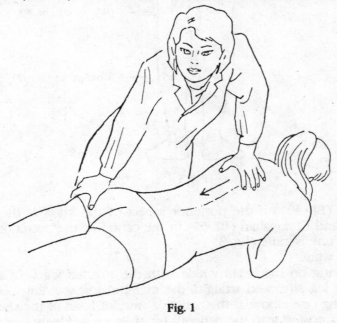

**Fig. 1**

197

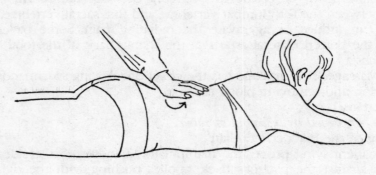

**Fig. 2**

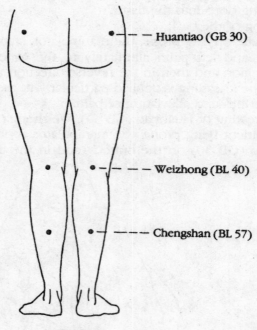

Huantiao (GB 30)

Weizhong (BL 40)

Chengshan (BL 57)

**Fig. 3**

trochanter, Weizhong (BL 40) on the posterior aspect of the knee, at the centre of the popliteal skin crease, and Chengshan (BL 57) in the centre of the posterior aspect of the shank, each for about one minute (fig. 3).

(4) Turning of the waist

With the patient lying on the healthy side with the affected leg bent at the hip and knee, and the healthy leg stretched straight, the manipulator, standing behind with the elbows bent and placing one elbow at the patient's anterior fossa of the shoulder and the other elbow at the area posterior to the patient's tip of ilium, suddenly turns the body 1-3 times by moving the two elbows in opposite directions with proper force. Usually there is a clear sound audible while turning the patient's waist (fig. 4). Thereafter, similar manipulation is performed on the healthy side.

(5) Pressing-kneading of Fengshi (GB 31), Yanglingquan (GB 34) and Jiexi (ST 41)

With the patient lying supine, the manipulator, standing to the side, applies pressing-kneading with the thumb tips to Fengshi (GB 31), on the lateral aspect of the thigh at the point where the tip of the middle finger touches the thigh when in standing position, Yanglingquan (GB 34), in the depression anterio-inferior to the capitulum of the fibula, and Jiexi (ST 41), in the depression in the centre of the ankle between the two tendons, each for one minute (fig. 5).

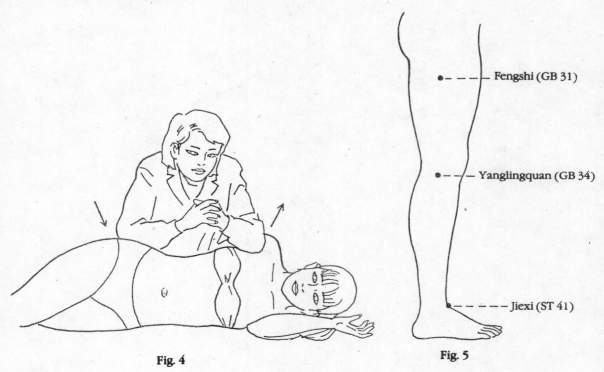

Fig. 4

Fengshi (GB 31)

Yanglingquan (GB 34)

Jiexi (ST 41)

Fig. 5

(6) Swaying of the lumbo-sacral region

With the patient lying supine, bending the hips and knees and holding the knees with both hands, the manipulator, supporting the patient's back with one hand and the knees with the other hand, asks the patient to sway the lumbo-sacral region to and fro for about one minute (fig. 6).

2. Self-massage

(1) Patting of the lumbo-sacral portion

Take a sitting position with the fingers closed and slightly bent, placing the palms on the lumbo-sacral region. Repeatedly pat the lumbo-sacral region for about three minutes, and then rub this region for two minutes (fig. 7).

199

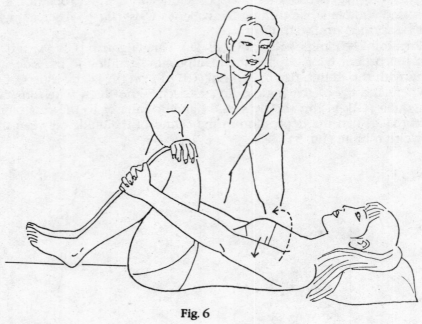

**Fig. 6**

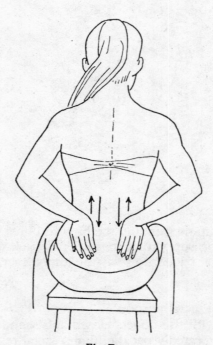

**Fig. 7**

(2) Pinching-grasping of the tender point of the affected limb

Take a sitting position. Pinch and grasp the tender point of the affected limb with the thumb and the other four fingers for 2-3 minutes.

(3) Extension of the knee in supine position

Lie supine with the knees extending straight. Slowly bend the knee and flex the hip and then extend (fig. 8). Repeatedly perform the exercise with the right and left knee alternately for about 1-2 minutes.

NB:

(1) It is important to rule out bone lesions before acupoint massage.

(2) The manipulation should be performed with appropriate force. It should be noted that improper manipulation may make the condition worse.

(3) Sleeping in a hard bed and keeping the lower back warm are recommended.

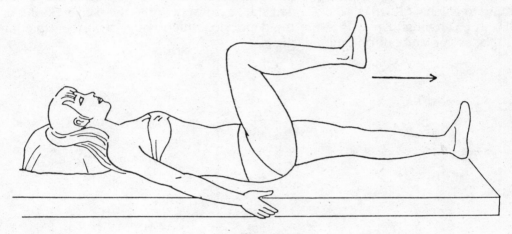

Fig. 8

## Systremma

Cause: Systremma, spasm of the gastrocnemius muscle, is often due to overfatigue of the lower limbs, traumatic injury, swimming or calcium deficit during pregnancy. It also frequently occurs in the aged who have general weakness, reduced functional activities and impaired blood circulation and have had exposure to cold.

Main Symptoms: Sudden spasm and rigidity of the gastrocnemius muscle with intolerable pain, inability to move and local bulging which is hard on palpation. The patient is often awakened from sleep by systremma.

Acupoint Massage: This massage has the effect of soothing the muscles, relieving spasm, promoting blood circulation and arresting pain.

[Manipulation]

*1. Massage by a family member*

(1) Point-pressing of Chengshan (BL 57) and Weizhong (BL 40)

With the patient lying prone, the manipulator, standing to the side, applies point-pressing to Chengshan (BL 57) in the centre of the posterior aspect of the shank, and Weizhong (BL 40) on the posterior aspect of the knee, at the centre of the popliteal skin crease, each for 1-2 minutes until there is a local feeling of distension and numbness radiating to the foot (fig. 1).

(2) Poking of the Achilles tendon

With the patient lying prone, the manipulator, standing to the side, applies pressing and poking with the thumb to the Achilles tendon for about one minute (fig. 2).

(3) Pushing-kneading of the shank

With the patient lying prone, the manipulator, standing to the side, applies pushing while kneading with the right and left palm alternately to the posterior aspect of the affected shank from the upper to the lower for about five minutes (fig. 3).

(4) Pressing-kneading of Xuehai (SP 10) and Yanglingquan (GB 34)

With the patient lying supine, the manipulator, standing to the side, applies pressing-kneading to Xuehai (SP 10) of the affected side, 2 *cun* superior to the medial border of the patella, and Yanglingquan (GB 34) in the depression anterio-inferior to the capitulum of the fibula, each for about one minute (fig. 4).

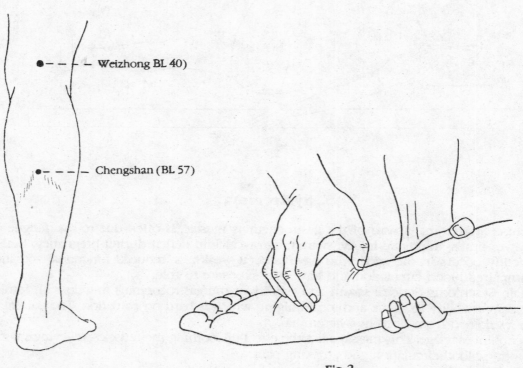

Fig. 1          Fig. 2

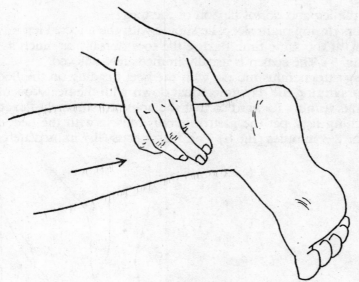

Fig. 3

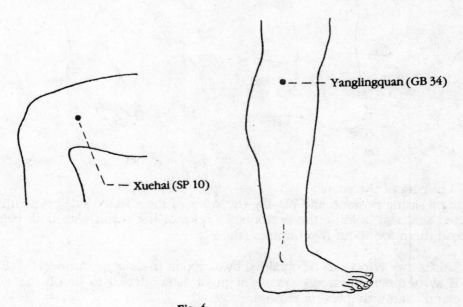

Xuehai (SP 10)

Yanglingquan (GB 34)

Fig. 4

203

### 2. Self-massage

(1) Stretching of the leg and dorsal flexion of the toes

If systremma occurs during night sleep, lie supine with the affected leg leaving the bed and stretch it straight, at the same time flexing the toes dorsally as much as possible for about 1-2 minutes (fig. 5). The spasm is usually immediately relieved.

(2) Patting of the gastrocnemius muscle with the heel treading on the floor

If systremma occurs during the day time, squat down with the heels touching the floor forcibly and the shanks leaning forward so that the ankle is extremely flexed, and at the same time half clenching fists, pat the gastrocnemius muscle with the heel of the palms somewhat forcibly for 2-3 minutes (fig. 6). The spasm is usually immediately relieved.

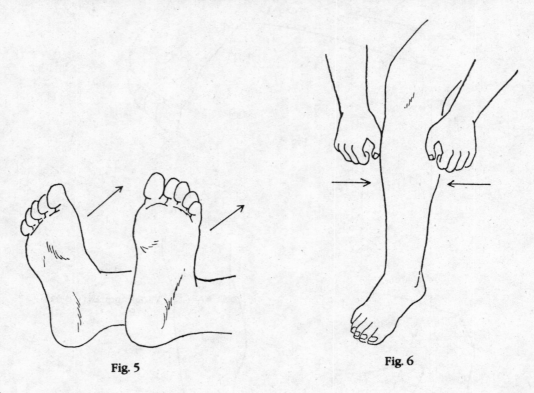

Fig. 5                                                Fig. 6

(3) Wringing of the shank

Taking a sitting position and placing the ankle of the affected side on the thigh of the unaffected side and holding the posterior muscles of the shank with both palms, wring and knead them for about five minutes (fig. 7).

NB:

(1) Satisfactory effect can be obtained by acupoint massage performed 1-2 times a day.

(2) If systremma repeatedly occurs at night, it is advised to lie on the side during sleeping and cautiously prevent exposure to cold.

(3) It is recommended to apply a hot water bag to the shanks in the aged during sleep at night.

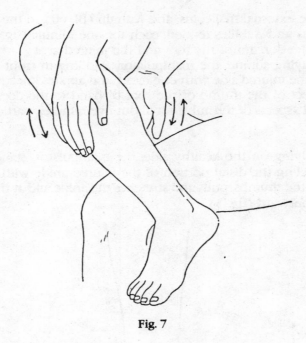

Fig. 7

## Sprain of the Ankle

Cause: A sprain of the ankle is a kind of soft tissue injury of the ankle joint, often due to slipping while walking, running, jumping, or going down the stairs or a hill, which makes one lose balance and causes excessive eversion or inversion of the foot, resulting in injury of the accessory ligaments of the ankle. Clinically, the ankle sprain caused by inversion with injury of the accessory ligament of the external malleolus is most common.

Main Symptoms: After injury there is swelling and pain of the ankle, and the patient is crippled or even unable to walk. Marked tenderness and local ecchymosis can be found. If the external malleolus is sprained, the pain is more marked when the foot is in inversion. If the internal malleolus is sprained, there is severe pain when the foot is in eversion and may be accompanied by laceration of the ligament. Sometimes, x-ray examination is necessary for the diagnosis.

Acupoint Massage: This massage activates blood circulation, removes ecchymosis, promotes the subsidence of swelling and relieves pain, and has satisfactory effect for treating simple sprain of the ligament.

[Manipulation]

1. Massage performed by a family member
(1) Point-pressing of Jiexi (ST 41), Qiuxu (GB 40) and Kunlun (BL 60)
With the patient lying supine, the manipulator, standing in front of the patient's feet, holds the injured ankle with one hand, and applies point-pressing with the thumb tip of the other hand to Jiexi (ST 41), on the anterior aspect of the ankle, at the midpoint of the transverse skin crease between the two tendons, Qiuxu (GB 40), in the depression

205

anterio-inferior to the external malleolus, and Kunlun (BL 60), in the depression between the external malleolus and Achilles tendon, each for one minute (fig. 1).

(2) Kneading of the dorsum of the foot and the injured area

With the patient lying supine, the manipulator, standing in front of the patient's feet, supports the heel of the injured side with one hand, and applies kneading softly and gently with the ventral aspect of the thumb or the root of hand to the dorsum of the foot and the medial and lateral aspects of the ankle for about five minutes, particularly to the injured area (fig. 2).

(3) Traction

With the patient lying on the healthy side, the manipulator, standing in front of the patient's feet and holding the distal portion of the injured ankle with both hands, presses the injured area with the thumbs, pulls and stretches the ankle and at the same time slightly turns it inward and outward (fig. 3).

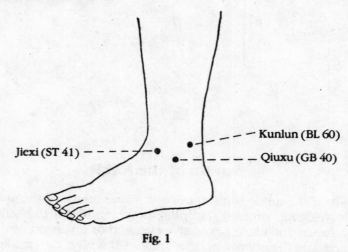

Kunlun (BL 60)

Jiexi (ST 41)

Qiuxu (GB 40)

Fig. 1

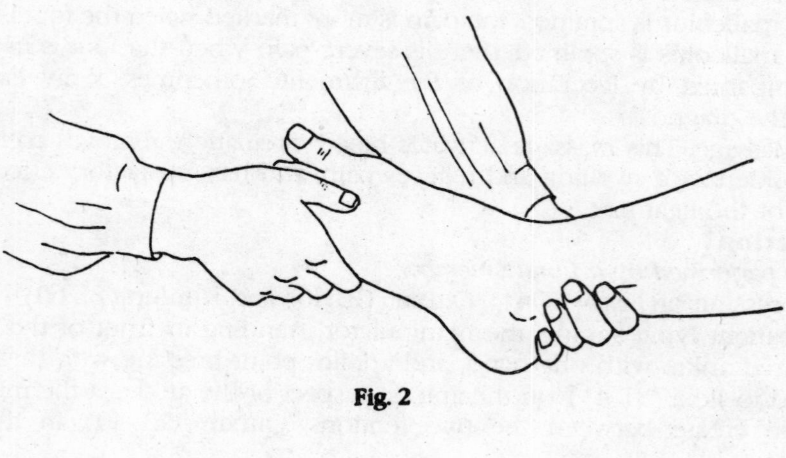

Fig. 2

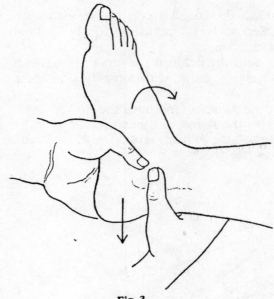

Fig. 3

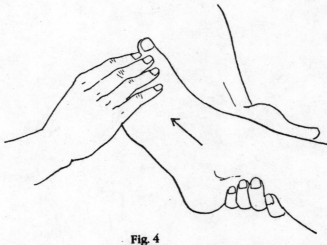

Fig. 4

(4) Dorsal extension of the ankle with flexion of the metatarsus

With the patient lying supine, the manipulator, standing in front of the patient's feet and supporting the heel of injured limb with one hand, holds the metatarsus and makes dorsal extension of the ankle as much as possible together with flexion and circular movements of the metatarsus for about one minute (fig. 4).

2. *Self-massage*

(1) Pushing of the shank of the injured limb

Take a sitting position. Push the lateral aspect of the shank with one palm from the upper to the lower (fig. 5). Repeat the manipulation for three minutes.

(2) Kneading of the tender point

Take a sitting position. Knead the ankle at the tender point with the thumb tip, using light force at first and then heavy together with active flexion and extension of the ankle for about three minutes.

(3) Pinching-grasping of the Achilles tendon of the injured limb

Take a sitting position with the shank of the injured limb on the knee of the healthy side. Repeatedly knead and grasp the Achilles tendon with the thumbs and fingers of both hands for about two minutes (fig. 6).

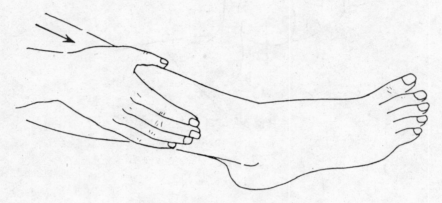

Fig. 5

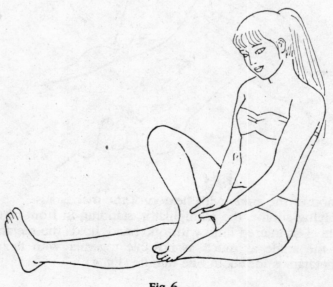

Fig. 6

NB:

(1) Acupoint massage once a day gives good effect for the treatment of simple sprain of ankle ligament.

(2) During the acute stage of the sprain, the patient is advised to have rest and elevation of the injured limb when sleeping.


# Pain in the Heel

Cause: A pain in the heel often occurs in the aged with weak constitution and obesity during walking or standing. It may be related to the senile degenerative change or a past injury that causes strain of the plantar fascia at its attachment to the calcaneus, not frequently accompanied by a spur at the anterior border of the tuberosity of the calcaneus, or related to aponeurositis secondary to a focal infection at some other part of the body.

Main Symptoms: A pain in the heel often occurs medio-inferior to the calcaneus during walking or standing, is more marked when treading the floor after getting up from lying or sitting, is alleviated by some activities, but is again aggravated if walking for too long. The pain may be precipitated by cold. On examination, there is local tenderness on the plantar aspect of the calcaneus at medial tuberosity. X-ray shows thickening of the soft tissue or calcaneal spur.

Acupoint Massage: This massage has the effect of soothing the tendons, activating blood circulation, promoting the subsidence of swelling and relieving pain.

[Manipulation]

*1. Massage performed by a family member*

(1) Point-pressing of Chengshan (BL 57) and Kunlun (BL 60)

With the patient lying prone, the manipulator, standing to the side and supporting the shank with one hand, applies point-pressing with the thumb of the other hand to Chengshan (BL 57), in the centre of posterior aspect of the leg between the two heads of the gastrocnemius muscle, and Kunlun (BL 60), in the depression between Achilles tendon and external malleolus, each for one minute (fig. 1).

(2) Kneading of the fundal portion of the heel

With the patient lying prone, the manipulator, sitting in front of the patient's feet and fixing the affected heel with one hand while placing the other palm on the fundal portion of the heel, applies kneading to this portion and its surroundings for about ten minutes (fig. 2).

(3) Pressing-poking of the tender point

With the patient lying prone, the manipulator, sitting in front of the patient's feet, fixes the affected heel with one hand, and applies pressing and poking repeatedly to the tender point of the affected area for about two minutes (fig. 3).

(4) Swaying-extending of the ankle

With the patient lying supine, the manipulator, sitting to the side and fixing the affected heel with one hand, holds the plantar portion of the foot and repeatedly makes dorsal extension, plantar flexion and clockwise swaying of the ankle for about one minute (fig. 4).

*2. Self-massage*

(1) Pinching-grasping of the shank and Achilles tendon

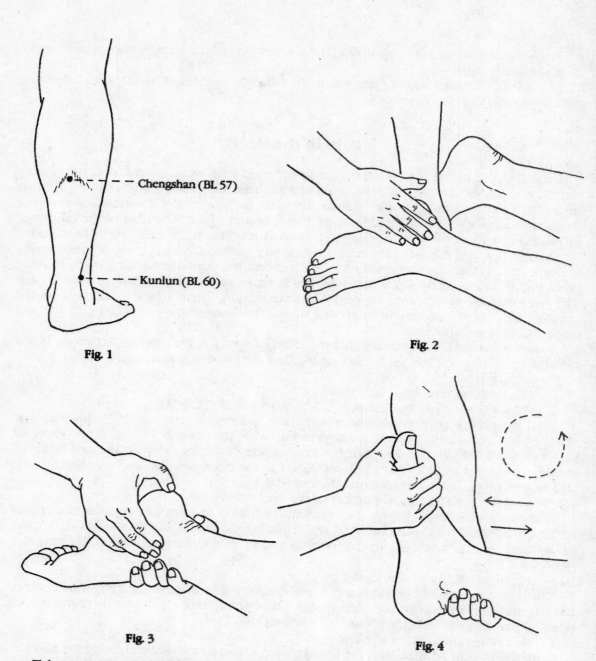

Chengshan (BL 57)

Kunlun (BL 60)

**Fig. 1**

**Fig. 2**

**Fig. 3**

**Fig. 4**

Take a sitting position. Pinch and grasp the posterior aspect of the shank with the thumbs and fingers of both hands from the upper shank to the heel (fig. 5). Repeat the manipulation for about two minutes.

(2) Rubbing of the heel

Take a sitting position with the shank of the affected side placed on the knee of the healthy side. Hold the dorsum of the affected foot with one hand and rub the heel and its surroundings with the other palm for about five minutes (fig. 6).

(3) Patting of the fundal portion of the heel

Take a sitting position with the shank of the affected side placed on the knee of the healthy side. Hold the dorsum of the affected foot with one hand, and pat the fundal

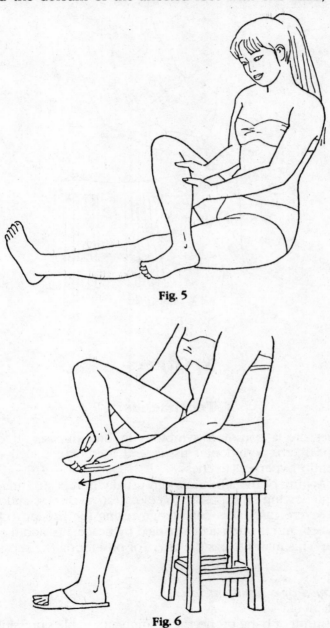

Fig. 5

Fig. 6

portion of the heel with the ulnar aspect of the other hand clenched into a fist (fig. 7). Perform the manipulation for about one minute.

NB:

(1) Perform the massage once daily or every other day.

(2) Immerse the feet in hot water for 30 minutes daily.

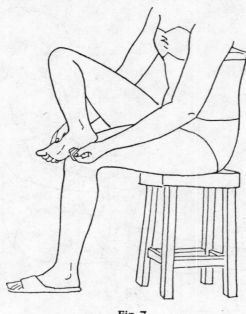

**Fig. 7**

# V. Others

## Toothaches

Cause: Toothaches are a common symptom in oral diseases. It occurs in various inflammations of the teeth, periodontal tissue and membrane, such as caries, pulpitis, periodontitis and dentin hypersensitiveness.

Main Symptoms: Aching of the affected tooth usually in repeated attacks. In mild cases, it only occurs during chewing or exposure to cold, heat, sweetness and sourness or when inhaling cool air; in severe cases, it is persistent, causing the patient to be unable to take food and have fast sleep, and is often accompanied by headaches and floating of the tooth.

Acupoint Massage: This massage has the effect of promoting the subsidence of swelling and relieving pain.

[Manipulation]

1. Massage performed by a family member

(1) Pressing of Hegu (LI 4)

With the patient sitting or lying prone, the manipulator applies pressing with the ventral aspect of the thumb to Hegu (LI 4) between the first and second metacarpal bones and at the midpoint of the radial aspect of the second metacarpal three minutes for each side (fig. 1). It is desirable to induce a feeling of local aching, distension, heaviness and numbness.

(2) Grasping of Jianjing (GB 21)

With the patient taking a sitting position, the manipulator, standing behind, applies grasping with both hands to Jianjing (GB 21) at the midpoint of the line joining the spinous process of the seventh thoracic vertebra and the acromion about one minute for each side (fig. 2).

(3) Kneading of the cheeks

With the patient lying supine, the manipulator, sitting behind the patient's head, applies kneading with the ventral aspect of the index, middle and ring fingers of both hands to the cheeks for about two minutes (fig. 3).

(4) Point-pressing of Jiache (ST 6)

With the patient lying supine, the manipulator, sitting behind the patient's head, applies point-pressing with the middle fingers to both Jiache (ST 6) simultaneously for about one minute (fig. 4). Jiache (ST 6) is located one finger's breadth anterior-superior to the angle of the mandible.

*2. Self-massage*

(1) Pressing-kneading of Fengchi (GB 20)

Take a sitting position. Apply pressing and kneading to both Fengchi (GB 20) with the thumb tips fixing the other fingers at the patient's occiput (fig. 5). Fengchi (GB 20) is located at the base of the skull, in the depression lateral to the sternocleidomastoid muscle and at the level of the lower border of the mastoid process.

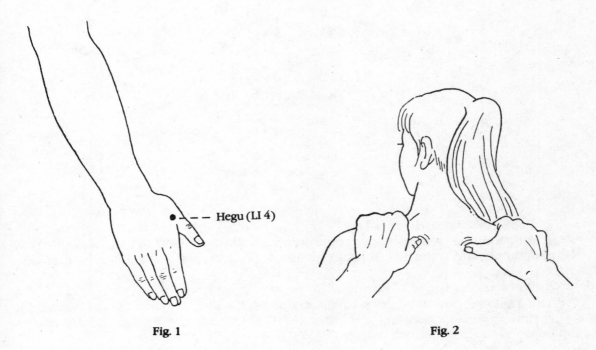

Fig. 1                                    Fig. 2

213

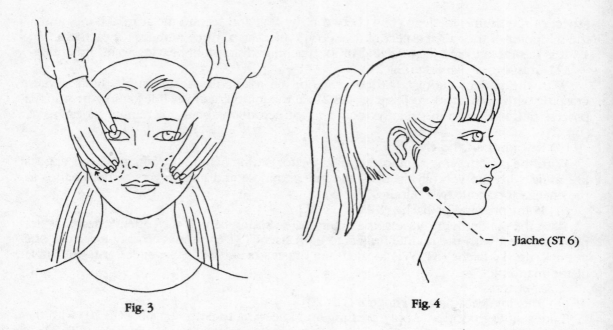

Fig. 3                                          Fig. 4

— Jiache (ST 6)

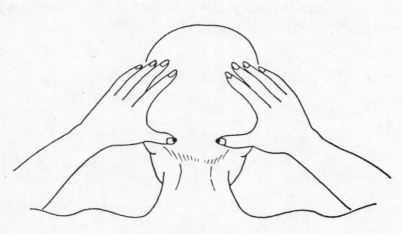

Fig. 5

(2) Point-pressing of Taixi (KI 3)

Sit with the legs crossed. Apply point-pressing with the thumb tips to Taixi (KI 3) at the midpoint between the medial malleolus and Achilles tendon, two minutes for each side (fig. 6).

(3) Pushing-pressing of Xiaguan (ST 7)

Take a sitting position. Apply pushing and pressing with the thumb tip to Xiaguan (ST 7) in the depression between the mandibular notch and the inferior border of the zygomatic arch for about one minute (fig. 7).

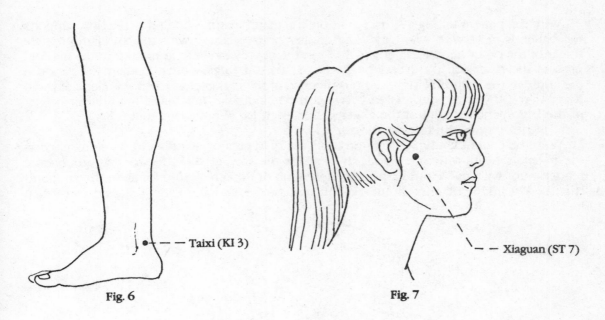

Taixi (KI 3)

Xiaguan (ST 7)

Fig. 6                                  Fig. 7

NB:

(1) Acupoint massage once in the morning and in the evening may give beneficial support to the dentist's treatment.

(2) It is important to keep good oral hygiene, particularly by rinsing the mouth after meals and brushing the teeth in the morning and evening.

## Dysfunction of Temporomandibular Joint

Cause: The temporomandibular joint is the only joint of the face that can move. It is composed of the glenoid cavity of the temporal bone, condyloid process of the mandible, a fibrocartilaginous disc, ligaments of the joint capsule and the masseter. Its dysfunction is often related to malocclusion, hypodontia, excessive abrasion, and a habit of unilateral chewing. Sometimes, dysfunction may be precipitated by direct trauma on the temporo-mandibular joint, yawning, chewing with violent force or exposure to cold that aggravates an injury of the temporomandibular joint and its surrounding muscles, tendons and nerves.

Main Symptoms: There is local aching when the mouth is open or closed, sometimes snapping can be heard during the movements of the mandibular joint. In severe cases, there is difficulty in opening the mouth and occluding, and aching, distension and weakness of the masseter. The dysfunction often occurs unilaterally with marked local tenderness.

Acupoint Massage: This massage has the effect of soothing the muscles and ligaments, relieving spasm and pain.

[Manipulation]

1. Massage performed by a family member

(1) Point-pressing of Yifeng (TE 17), Jiache (ST 6) and Xiaguan (ST 7) of the affected side

215

With the patient taking a sitting position, the manipulator, standing to the side, supports the patient's head with one hand, and applies point-pressing with the tip of the middle finger of the other hand to Yifeng (TE 17), in the depression anterio-inferior to the mastoid process and posterior to the earlobe, Jiache (ST 6), one finger's breadth anterio-superior to the angle of the mandible or at the prominence of the masseter as the jaw is clenched, and Xiaguan (ST 7), in the depression between the mandibular notch and the inferior border of the zygomatic arch, all of the affected side, each for about one minute (fig. 1).

(2) Kneading of the face on the affected side

With the patient taking a sitting position, the manipulator, standing to the side, supports the patient's head with one hand, and kneads the face of the affected side around the tender point with the ventral aspect of the thumb of the other hand for about five minutes (fig. 2). The manipulation should be soft and gentle, and the patient should feel warm locally.

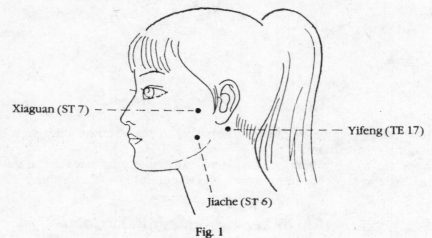

**Fig. 1**

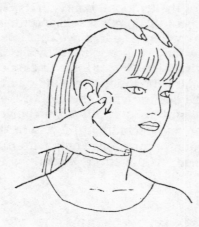

**Fig. 2**

(3) Swaying of the mandible

With the patient sitting with the occiput leaning against the wall, the manipulator, supporting the patient's mandible with hands on both sides, advises the patient to open the mouth and relax the temporomandibular joint, slowly swaying the patient's mandible upward, downward, rightward and leftward for about one minute (fig. 3).

2. *Self-massage*

(1) Kneading of the mandibular articulation of the affected side

Take a sitting position. Apply kneading with the ventral aspect of the index, middle and ring fingers to the mandibular articulation and its surrounding tissues of the affected side for about two minutes (fig. 4).

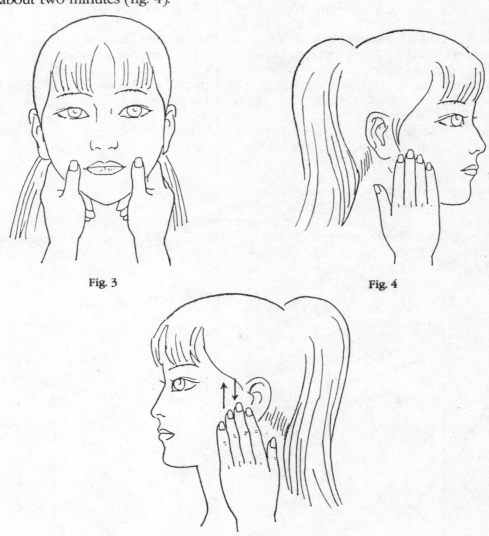

Fig. 3

Fig. 4

Fig. 5

(2) Rubbing beside the ear

Take a sitting position. Repeatedly rub the area anterior and posterior to the auricle with the index and middle fingers (exerting force particularly with the middle finger) for about two minutes (fig. 5).

NB:

(1) Cold stimulation and chewing hard food should be avoided during the massage treatment.

(2) A local hot compress is recommended.

## Tinnitus with Impaired Hearing

Cause: Tinnitus with impairment of hearing is a common symptom in auditory diseases. It often occurs in neurasthenia, anemia, hypertension, hypotension, Meniere's syndrome or results from the stimulation of noise, anger or fright.

Main Symptoms: A ringing in the ear(s) of various pitches and intensities, particularly marked in quiet circumstances, often accompanied by impaired hearing. Tinnitus occurs more frequently in the aged.

Acupoint Massage: This massage has the effect of removing obstruction from the meridians and collaterals, stopping the ringing in the ear(s) and promoting recovery of hearing.

**[Manipulation]**

*1. Massage performed by a family member*

(1) Kneading at the auricular region

With the patient lying supine, the manipulator, sitting behind the patient's head, applies kneading with the ventral aspect of the index, middle and ring fingers around the ear of the affected side(s), particularly near the tragus and earlobe (fig. 1). The manipulation is repeated for about three minutes.

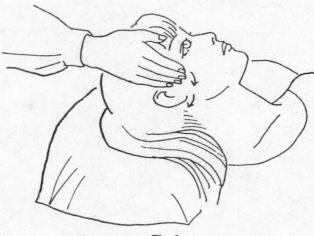

**Fig. 1**

218

(2) Pressing-kneading of Yifeng (TE 17)

With the patient lying supine, the manipulator, sitting behind the patient's head, applies pressing and kneading with the tip of the middle finger to Yifeng (TE 17) in the depression anterior to the mastoid process and posterior to the earlobe for about one minute (fig. 2).

(3) Point-pressing of Tinggong (SI 19)

With the patient lying supine, the manipulator, sitting behind the patient's head, applies point-pressing with the tip of the middle finger to Tinggong (SI 19) in the depression anterior to the tragus and posterior to the condylar process of the mandible for about one minute (fig. 3).

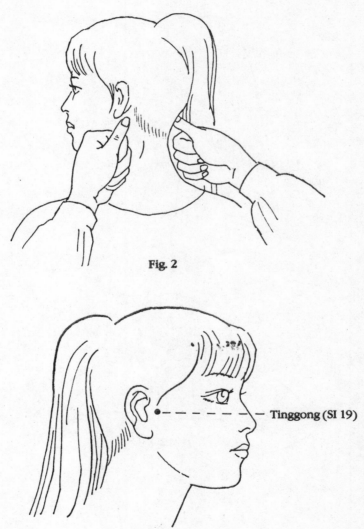

Fig. 2

Tinggong (SI 19)

Fig. 3

## 2. Self-massage

(1) Pinching-grasping of the auricle

Take a sitting position. Slowly pinch, grasp, lift and pull the auricle, particularly the earlobe and apex, with the index and middle fingers for about one minute (fig. 4).

(2) Pressing of the earhole

Take a sitting position. Press the earholes with the centre of the palms, gently at first, then with force, and then suddenly relax (fig. 5). Repeat the manipulation 3-5 times.

(3) Tapping of Fengchi (GB 20)

Take a sitting position. Slightly bending the palms and pressing the earholes with the

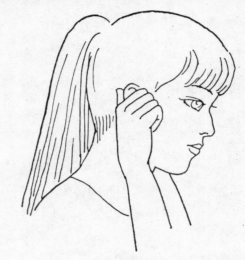

**Fig. 4**

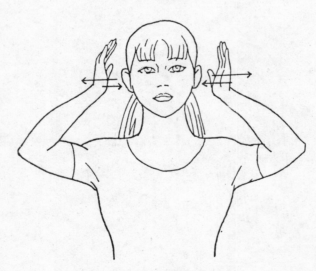

**Fig. 5**

centre of the palms and placing the middle fingers on the occiputs, tap the base of the skull at Fengchi (GB 20) with the tip of the index fingers for about one minute (fig. 6).

(4) Rubbing beside the ear

Take a sitting position. Apply rubbing beside the auricle with the ventral aspect of the index and middle fingers up and down repeatedly for about one minute (fig. 7).

(5) Pressing-kneading of Shenshu (BL 23)

Take a sitting position. Clench the fists and apply pressing with the interphalangeal joint of the thumbs to Shenshu (BL 23), 1.5 *cun* lateral to the midpoint between the spinous processes of the second and third lumbar vertebrae, for about two minutes (fig. 8).

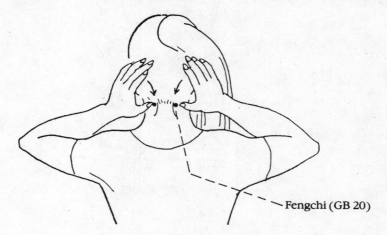

Fengchi (GB 20)

Fig. 6

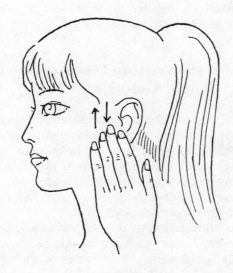

Fig. 7

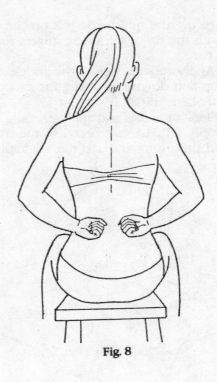

Fig. 8

NB:

(1) It is advised to perform acupoint massage twice a day, in the morning and in the evening, with gentle and soft manipulation.

(2) The patient should have a regular lifestyle with a calm mood and appropriate alteration of work with rest and recreation.

## Acupoint Massage for Preventing Diseases and Guaranteeing Longevity

Acupoint massage is a health maintenance method developed by the Chinese people and Chinese medical doctors in their centuries-long struggle against diseases. It has a history of more than one thousand years. It is not only a part of the valuable heritage of traditional Chinese medicine, but also a component of physical therapy and rehabilitation practised at present. Learning self-acupoint massage and appropriately applying the massage in accordance with one's health conditions is very helpful for the aged to protect health, prevent diseases and guarantee longevity.

Self-massage which gives stimulation to the acupoints and peripheral nerves is chiefly aimed at promoting blood and lymph circulation and tissue metabolism, regulating the cerebral cortical function and enhancing the activities of the central nervous system and visceral organs. Therefore, it can be used to improve the constitution, prevent diseases and guarantee longevity.

## [Manipulation]

(1) Stroking of the face

Rub the palms warm, then stroke the face with the palms beside the nose, around the orbits, along the forehead and near the ears in circular movements like washing the face for about one minute (fig. 1).

(2) Kneading of the head

Slightly bending the fingers of both hands and keeping them separate, insert them in the hair on the scalp and gently knead the scalp as if washing the hair (fig. 2). Continue the kneading for one minute.

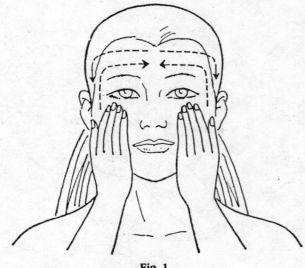

Fig. 1

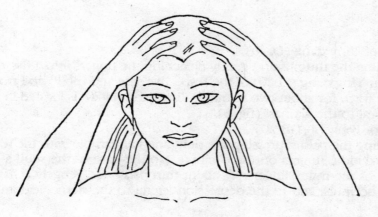

Fig. 2

(3) Rubbing of the nape

Crossing the fingers of the right and left hands and holding the nape with both hands, bend the head somewhat backward and then rub the nape to and fro with the hands for about two minutes (fig. 3).

(4) Kneading of Taiyang (EX-HN 5)

Placing the hypothenar prominences of the right and left palms on the respective temporal at Taiyang (EX-HN 5) in the depression lateral to the external end of the eyebrow and the external canthus of the eye, make clockwise kneading for about thirty seconds and then counterclockwise kneading for another thirty seconds (fig. 4).

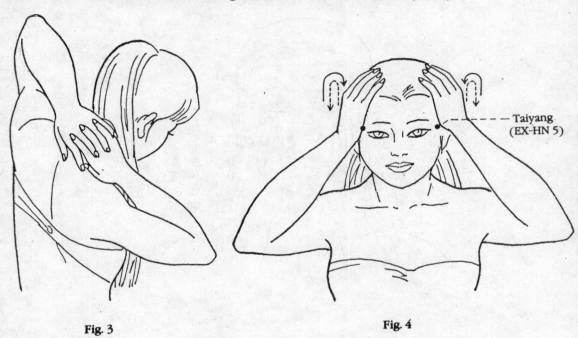

Fig. 3                              Fig. 4

(5) Rubbing of Yingxiang (LI 20)

Slightly bending the thumbs and gently clenching the fingers into a fist, place the right and left thumb at Yingxiang (LI 20) of the respective side and rub to and fro along the ala nasi with proper force for about two minutes. Yingxiang (LI 20) is located in the nasolabial fold, 0.5 *cun* lateral to the ala nasi (fig. 5).

(6) Tapping of Fengchi (GB 20)

Slightly bending the palms, pressing the right and left earhole with the respective palm and placing the middle fingers on the occiputs, tap the base of the skull at Fengchi (GB 20) with the tip of the index fingers for about thirty seconds. Fengchi (GB 20) is located posterior to the occiputs, and in the depression lateral to the sternocleidomastoid muscle (fig. 6).

(7) Vibrating of the ear

Extend the fingers and press the right and left earhole with the respective palm. Make

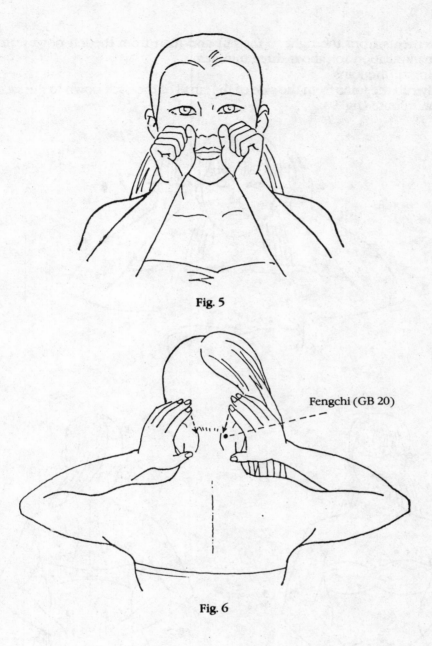

Fig. 5

Fengchi (GB 20)

Fig. 6

vibration and close pressing to the earholes, and then suddenly relax (fig. 7). Repeat the manipulation 3-5 times.

(8) Stroking of the abdomen

Placing the right palm on the umbilicus and the left palm against the dorsum of the right hand, stroke the abdomen with the overlapped hands around the umbilicus in

circular movements from the right to the left and then from the left downward (fig. 8).
Repeat the manipulation for about three minutes.

(9) Rubbing of the loins

Repeatedly rub the loins from the side of the small of the back down to the sacral region for about one minute (fig. 9).

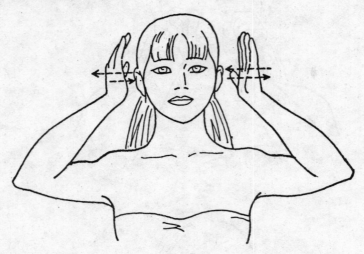

Fig. 7

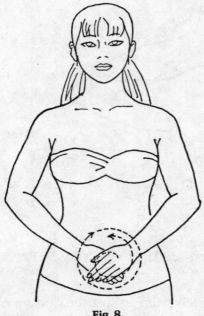

Fig. 8

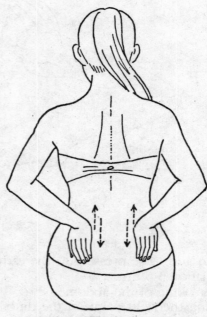

Fig. 9

(10) Turning of the knee

Placing the feet on the floor close together in parallel, and slightly squatting down with the palms on the knees, turn the knees rightward in circular movements for thirty seconds and then leftward for another thirty seconds (fig. 10).

(11) Pressing of Zusanli (ST 36)

Apply pressing and kneading with the right and left thumb to Zusanli (ST 36) of the respective side for about one minute. Zusanli (ST 36) is located 3 *cun* inferior to the lateral aspect of the knee and one finger's breadth lateral to the tibial crest (fig. 11).

(12) Rubbing of Yongquan (KI 1)

Placing the right foot on the left thigh, the right palm closely against the right knee, and the hypothenar prominence of the left hand on Yongquan (KI 1), in the centre of the sole of the foot between the second and third metatarsals, rub the right knee and

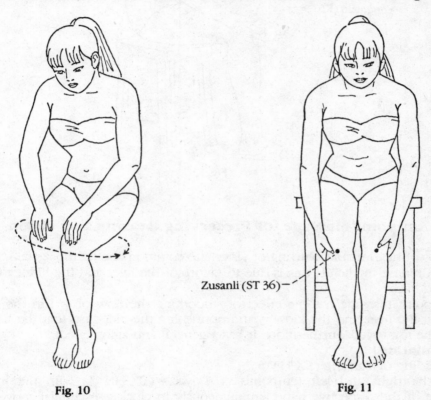

Zusanli (ST 36)—

Fig. 10                              Fig. 11

Yongquan (KI 1) simultaneously for about one minute (fig. 12). Then perform similar manipulation on the left foot.

NB:

(1) Self-massage in the morning and in the evening is effective for preventing diseases and treating diseases at the early stage.

(2) The key points are general relaxation, concentration of the mind, and gentle and soft manipulation with proper force. Inadequate force cannot give appropriate stimulation.

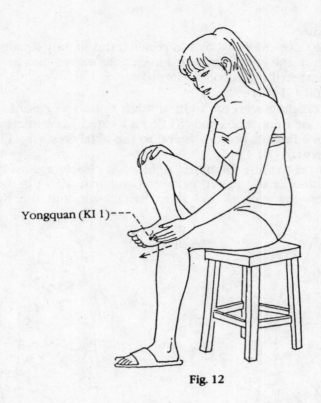

Yongquan (KI 1)

Fig. 12

## Acupoint Massage for Preserving Hearing and Vision

Hardness of hearing and blurring of vision are common among the aged. According to traditional Chinese medicine, this is due to failure of the liver and the kidney to nourish the ears and eyes.

Self-acupoint massage has the effect of smoothing the flow of *qi* i in the meridians, replenishing the liver and the kidney, and nourishing the blood, so that the hearing and vision can be improved. Furthermore, it has a general anti-aging effect.

**[Manipulation]**

(1) Kneading of Taiyang (EX-HN 5)

Knead the right and left temporals at Taiyang (EX-HN 5) with the hypothenar prominence of the respective hand simultaneously in clockwise circular movements for thirty seconds and then in counterclockwise circular movements for another thirty seconds (fig. 1). Taiyang (EX-HN 5) is located in the depression one finger's breadth lateral to the external end of the eyebrow and the external canthus of the eye.

(2) Pressing of Jingming (BL 1)

Press both Jingming (BL 1) with the tips of the middle fingers simultaneously for about one minute. Jingming (BL 1) is located in the depression 0.1 *cun* superior to the inner canthus of the eye (fig. 2).

(3) Pushing of the orbits

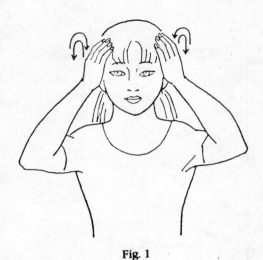

Fig. 1

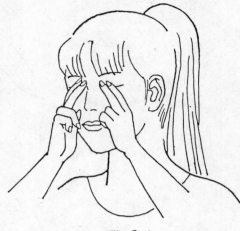

Fig. 2

Half close the eyes. Apply pushing to both orbits with the ventral aspect of the index and middle fingers of both hands simultaneously, starting from the inner canthus of the eyes along the lower border of the orbits to the outer canthus of the eyes and then back to the inner canthus along the upper border of the orbits (fig. 3). Repeat the pushing for two minutes.

(4) Pressing-kneading of Shenshu (BL 23)

Slightly bend the thumbs and gently clench the fingers into fists. Apply pressing and kneading with the dorsal articular prominence of the thumbs to Shenshu (BL 23) of the respective side simultaneously for about one minute. Shenshu (BL 23) is located 1.5 *cun* lateral to the midpoint between the spinous processes of the second and third lumbar vertebrae (fig. 4).

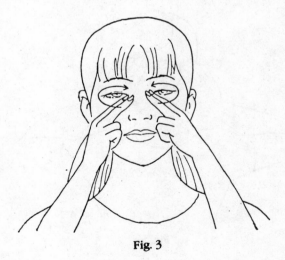

Fig. 3

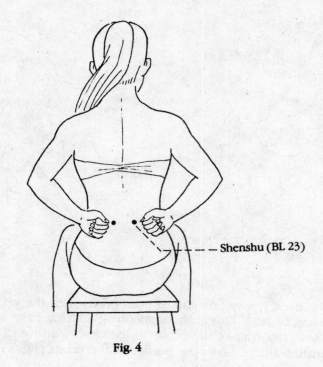

Shenshu (BL 23)

Fig. 4

(5) Tapping of Fengchi (GB 20)

Pressing the right and left earhole with the respective palm and placing the middle fingers on the occiputs, tap the base of the skull at Fengchi (GB 20) with the tip of the index fingers for about one minute. Fengchi (GB 20) is located in the depression inferior to the occipital bone and lateral to the sternocleidomastoid muscle.

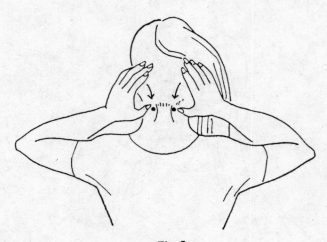

Fig. 5

(6) Point-pressing of Tinggong (SI 19)

Apply point-pressing with the middle fingers to right and left Tinggong (SI 19) simultaneously for about one minute. Tinggong (SI 19) is located on the face in the depression anterior to the tragus as the mouth is open (fig. 6).

(7) Pinching-grasping of the auricle

Placing the thumb and index finger of the right and left hand on the respective auricle, apply repeatedly pinching and grasping for about two minutes to the auricle from the posterior to the anterior together with gently lifting and pulling of the earlobe and apex (fig. 7).

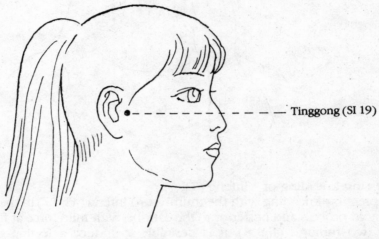

Tinggong (SI 19)

**Fig. 6**

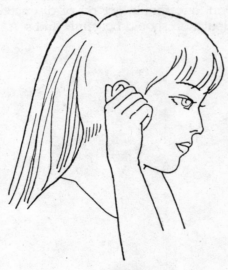

**Fig. 7**

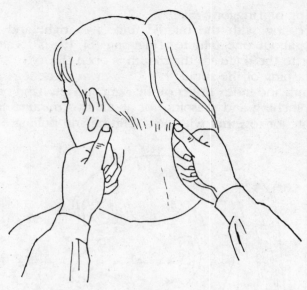

**Fig. 8**

(8) Pressing-kneading of Yinfeng (TE 17)

Apply pressing-kneading with the thumbs to Yinfeng (TE 17) in the depression anterior to the mastoid process and posterior to the earlobe, with mild force at first and then heavier for about two minutes (fig. 8). It is desirable to induce a feeling of local aching and distension.

NB:

(1) Perform self-massage every day in the morning and in the evening.

(2) During the manipulation, one should get rid of distractions and concentrate the mind on the hands. The manipulation should be gentle and soft.

中国家庭经穴按摩

王传贵

\*

外文出版社出版

（中国北京百万庄路24号）

邮政编码100037

北京外文印刷厂印刷

1992年（16开）第一版

1994年第二次印刷

（英）

ISBN 7－119－01439－O／R.78（外）

06820

14－E－2696(P)